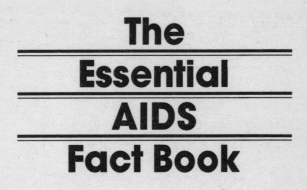

The
Essential
AIDS
Fact Book

Also by Paul Harding Douglas and Laura Pinsky

The Essential HIV Treatment Fact Book

Published by POCKET BOOKS

The Essential AIDS Fact Book

NEWLY REVISED AND UPDATED

by
Paul Harding Douglas and Laura Pinsky

Preface by Mathilde Krim, Ph.D.,
Founding Co-chair,
American Foundation for AIDS Research

POCKET BOOKS

New York   London   Toronto   Sydney   Tokyo   Singapore

An *Original* Publication of POCKET BOOKS

POCKET BOOKS, a division of Simon & Schuster Inc.
1230 Avenue of the Americas, New York, NY 10020

Library of Congress Cataloging-in-Publication Data

Douglas, Paul Harding.
    The essential AIDS fact book / Paul Harding Douglas and Laura
Pinsky; preface by Mathilde Krim. Newly revised and updated.
        p.   cm.
    Includes bibliographical references.
    ISBN 0-671-55287-2
    1. AIDS (Disease)—Popular works.   I. Pinsky, Laura.   II. Title.
RC607.A26D68   1996
616.97'92— dc20   95-48199
                                                                              CIP

First Pocket Books trade paperback printing May 1996

10   9   8   7   6   5   4   3

POCKET and colophon are registered trademarks of
Simon & Schuster Inc.

Printed in the U.S.A.

ACKNOWLEDGMENTS

The fourth edition was prepared with the assistance of Michael Giordano, MD, and Theo Smart.

The authors would like to thank the following individuals and organizations for their help and support: Priscilla Alexander; Kevin Armington; Donald Armstrong, MD; Jody Asnis; Michael Barr; Kevin Berrill; Bernard Bihari, MD; John Bloomfield; Christine Bratton; Michael Callen; Richard G. Carlson, MD; Kate Cauley, PhD; Alden Cohen; Columbia Lesbian Bisexual & Gay Coalition; Columbia Psychological Counseling Service; Jack DeHovitz, MD; Tina Dobesevage, MD; Colette Smith Douglas; Paul Wolff Douglas; Jill Eden, MBA, MPH; Richard Eichler, PhD; Alexa Freeman, JD; Bob Friedman; Gay Men's Health Crisis; Kathleen Gilberd; Richard Glendon, MD; Judy Greenspan; Ted Hammett, PhD; Douglas Henwood; Scott Holmberg, MD; Milton Horowitz, MD; Rose Inman, FNP; Jonathan Jacobs, MD; John S. James; the Jones family; Donald Kaplan, PhD; Martha Katz, MD; Richard Keeling, MD; James Kellogg, JD; John Kender, PhD; Robert Kertzner, MD; Robert Klein, MD; Lambda Legal Defense and Education Fund; Michael Lange, MD; Jeffrey Laurence, MD; Gary Ledet; Elena Levine, MD; Laura Long, MS; Lynne McArthur; Meade Morgan, MD; Joseph P. Mullinix; Jody Newman; Stacey Oliker, PhD; Florence Pinsky; Juliette Pinsky; Charles Pinsky; Suki Ports; Barbara Prisco; Amado Punsalong, PhD; Michel Radomisli, PhD; Lisa Robinson, NP; Bill Rold; Jill Rubin, CSW; Edith Springer, CSW; Joe Stonehouse; Susan Tross, PhD; Dan Tsing, MD, PhD; John Ward, MD; Lois R. Whelk; Ron Winchel, MD; and Jerry Wolbert, FNP.

Special thanks to Dan Altilio, Sarah Chinn, Michael Dowling, Bruce Francis, Gerard Ilaria, Jason Klein, David Klotz, Maria McKenna, Wayne Steward, Anita Tierney, Diane Watkin, and all the volunteers of the Columbia Gay Health Advocacy Project.

The authors particularly thank the following people, who generously gave their time to review the content of sections of this book:

Charles A. Barber

Mark Barnes, JD

William Flanagan, LLB, DEA, LLM

Barry Gingell, MD

Thaddeus Grimes-Gruczka

Karl Hoffman, MD

Donald Kotler, MD

Mathilde Krim, PhD

Craig Metroka, MD, PhD

Robert Padgug, PhD

Martha Rogers, MD

Charles Schable, MS

Mark Scherzer, Esq.

Joseph Sonnabend, MD

Kendall Thomas, JD

Daniel William, MD

Any errors that remain are the sole responsibility of the authors.

For PHD with my best love always.

LP

CONTENTS

PREFACE

The Essential AIDS Fact Book is exactly what its title says it is: a book in which anyone can find an accurate description of the essential facts—biological, medical, psychological, social, and legal—of HIV infection and AIDS in our society. Bibliographical references, usually absent from books for lay readers, refer to sources of information and suggest further useful readings.

Paul Harding Douglas, Laura Pinsky, and the Columbia University Health Service must be thanked for their evident humane concern for all at risk of, or afflicted by, HIV infection or AIDS, to whom they provide thoughtful, considerate, yet sober, and practical advice. They are also to be commended for their grasp of the complex, dynamic processes at play in the unfolding epidemic and their ability to write about them in a lucid and concise way.

This book should be a "must read" for all college-age youth and sexually active adults.

Mathilde Krim, PhD
Associate research scientist, St. Luke's/Roosevelt Hospital Center and College of Physicians and Surgeons, Columbia University*
Founding co-chair, American Foundation for AIDS Research*

---

*Affiliations listed for identification purposes only.

INTRODUCTION

It is hard to realize that we are now more than fifteen years into the AIDS epidemic. An illness that once seemed so mysterious has now been largely defined as to its modes of transmission, immunologic effects, natural history, and pathophysiology; but advances in treatment are still measured as tiny fractions of longer life, there is no vaccine to prevent the illness, and no one has been cured. Despite the millions of cases worldwide and the millions spent to define and defeat the disease, it is estimated that by the year 2000, 8 million people worldwide will have died of AIDS.

What can be done? Research goes on and hope lives on. AIDS has become a part of our culture—the epidemic is rendered in books, film, music, dance, and other art; but it is most dramatically felt in the lives of people living with AIDS, and living with people living with AIDS. Portraying the illness in a play or in a movie has not tamed the plague and should not distance us from it. It is not taken care of, it is not going away, it is all around us.

This small book will tell you what you need to know about AIDS. It is written by people who know what they're talking about and who have had experience in AIDS education and counseling. In writing this book they have had the help of a number of people associated with this university, and the information in this book has been distributed to the students and staff at Columbia.

While we recognize that some readers may be offended by the sexually explicit material in the Risk-Reduction Guidelines, this information must be included because its dissemination is at present the only way to limit the spread of the disease. The Health Service further recognizes that there are many strongly held views regarding appropriate sexual behavior of consenting adults and believes that each individual should carefully make decisions regarding sexual behavior for himself or herself.

The University Health Service strongly advises against the illegal use of intravenous drugs but has included cautions in this book to minimize health problems for those who do not accept our advice on drug use.

You should read this book carefully. It will tell you a great deal, and in clear language. It will also help you to better follow the dynamic and developing area of AIDS research. Most of all, it will give you some control in your life and relationships over one of the most serious public health problems the world and you as an individual have ever had to face.

Any proceeds that the university receives from this book will be used for health education and AIDS counseling.

Richard G. Carlson, MD
Director, Columbia University Health Service

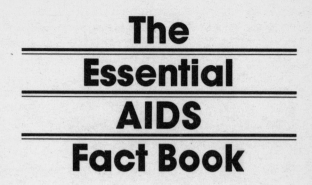

The
Essential
AIDS
Fact Book

1

Causes, Characteristics, and Transmission

In 1981, when the federal Centers for Disease Control (CDC) first began monitoring AIDS, the number of cases was small and little was known. As of June 1995, 476,899 cases of AIDS had been reported in the United States.[1] At least another 231,000 people in the United States are living with HIV infection. As of 1995, there were estimated to be 4.5 million cases of AIDS worldwide and 19.5 million cases of HIV infection.[2] Because researchers have spent years studying the vast amount of data associated with these cases, certain aspects of AIDS are now well understood.

HIV INFECTION AND AIDS

AIDS is an illness that damages a person's ability to fight off disease, leaving the body open to attack from ordinarily innocuous infections and some forms of cancers. *AIDS* stands for *A*cquired *I*mmuno*D*eficiency *S*yndrome. AIDS is not a single disease: rather, it is a constellation of symptoms caused by infections and/or cancers, primarily due to disruption of the immune system by an underlying viral infection. *Pneumocystis carinii* pneumonia (PCP) has been the most common cause of death in people with AIDS in the United States. Other frequent infections are cytomegalovirus (CMV), *Mycobacterium avium* complex (MAC), and crytosporidiosis. Other serious medical problems are lymphoma, Kaposi's sarcoma (KS), loss of lean body mass (wasting), and neurological difficulties.[3]

HIV Damages Various Cells

AIDS is caused by a virus called HIV, which stands for *H*uman *I*mmunodeficiency *V*irus. This virus infects certain types of white blood cells: principally CD4 cells (also called helper cells or T4 cells) and monocytes/macrophages. CD4 cells and macrophages both have important functions in the immune system. The disruption of the function of these cells lies at the heart of the immunodeficiency that characterizes AIDS. The virus also infects and causes damage to other types of cells: damage to the lining of the intestine[4] may contribute to wasting (severe weight loss); damage to nerve cells[5, 6] sometimes causes dementia, peripheral neuropathy, or other neurological problems.

Spectrum of HIV Infection

AIDS is a diagnostic category constructed by the CDC. Its definition has changed over time. Since 1993, *AIDS* has been defined as "a specific group of diseases or conditions which are indicative of severe immunosuppression related to infection with the human immunodeficiency virus (HIV)."[7] People who fit the CDC's criteria are described as having "CDC-defined AIDS" or "full-blown" AIDS.

We will use the term *HIV disease* to mean the full spectrum of conditions caused by HIV infection, including asymptomatic HIV infection, symptomatic infection, and AIDS.

Some HIV-Infected People Develop AIDS

A percentage of HIV-infected people develop AIDS each year. Scientific predictions have varied regarding the proportion of infected people who will fall seriously ill in the long term. Without new treatment, the majority of infected people will develop AIDS within fifteen years.[8] However, some people who have been infected this long remain healthy. Currently the average time from infection to AIDS is eight to fifteen years. Treatment advances may change these predictions dramatically.

Other Factors May Contribute to Development of Illness

It is not known if some people are more easily infected than others, nor why some people who are infected with HIV have become ill while others have remained healthy. Some researchers think that other conditions, called co-factors, may contribute to the development of the more serious forms of HIV infection. Others suggest that different strains of the virus or hereditary factors play a role.

Opportunistic Infections and Cancers Are Primary Causes of Death from AIDS

If HIV infection progresses, it can cause serious damage to the immune system. As a result, certain cancers may appear and ordinarily harmless infections may be reactivated, causing serious illness.[9] These infections are referred to as opportunistic, since, although latently present in most people, they only cause illness in people with immune impairment. Opportunistic infections and cancers are currently the cause of most of the deaths in AIDS patients.

Organisms that commonly cause opportunistic infections in people with AIDS are listed in the following table:

	Organism	Diseases Caused
Parasites	Pneumocystis carinii (may be a fungus)	Pneumonia
	Toxoplasma gondii	Diseases of the central nervous system
	Cryptosporidia	Diarrhea, wasting
	Microsporidia	Diarrhea, wasting
	Candida	Thrush, esophagitis
	Cryptococcus	Meningitis
	Histoplasma	Pulmonary, systemic disease
Bacteria	Mycobacterium tuberculosis	Tuberculosis
	Mycobacterium avium	Disseminated disease
	Salmonella, Shigella, Campylobacter, C. difficile	Gastrointestinal disease (including diarrhea, colitis, and wasting)
	Streptococcus, H. Influenza, Staphylococcus, Pseudomonas	Bacterial pneumonia, sinusitis, skin and bone infections
Viruses	Adenovirus	Gastrointestinal disease
	B19 parvovirus	Anemia
	Cytomegalovirus	Retinitis, colitis, encephalitis
	Herpes	Herpes, shingles, chicken pox
	Human papilloma virus (HPV)	Cervical dysplasia, genital and anal warts
	JC virus	PML (brain disease)

The most frequent cancers are Kaposi's sarcoma (a cancer of the linings of blood vessels) and, less often, lymphoma (cancers of the lymph nodes). Although Kaposi's sarcoma can be fatal, it has a relatively slow course, and most people with Kaposi's sarcoma eventually develop other opportunistic diseases that are more life-threatening. There is some scientific question as to whether Kaposi's sarcoma is actually a form of cancer.[10]

Gastrointestinal and Nervous System Involvement

Various opportunistic infections and possibly HIV itself can damage the lining of the intestine. This interferes with the absorption of nourishment causing the loss of lean tissue such as muscle. This wasting further weakens the body's ability to fight disease and itself can be fatal.[11]

HIV can damage the central nervous system (CNS), including the brain. Some opportunistic infections, particularly *cryptococcus*, *toxoplasmosis*, and progressive multifocal leukoencephalopathy (PML) also cause diseases of the CNS.[12] Central nervous system infections are a common manifestation of AIDS. Problems range from very mild (for example, minor problems with memory)[13] to very severe (for example, dementia or delirium).[14] However, studies show that serious organically caused mental-problem symptoms generally develop after physical symptoms and relatively late in the course of the disease.[15] Peripheral nervous system problems (peripheral neuropathy) frequently occur in HIV disease and are caused by a number of factors including medication, HIV itself, and other infections. The symptoms can range from tingling in the fingers to numbness or pain in arms and legs that interferes with functioning.[16]

TREATMENT IMPROVING

To control the worst consequences of HIV infection it is necessary not only to stop the growth of the virus, but also to repair the immune system, treat or prevent the various opportunistic infections and cancers, and reverse the bodily wasting sometimes associated with AIDS. Effective therapy for HIV disease may have to be a combination of several different treatments. Developments in treatment have allowed HIV-infected people to stay healthy and live longer.

Many AIDS-related cancers and opportunistic infections are fully or partially treatable with medication. Treatment and prevention have improved radically in the last few years and are primarily responsible for increased life expectancy. PCP, which has been responsible for over 60% of AIDS deaths, is preventable in the majority of cases.[17]

PCP is still the most common cause of death from AIDS because many people are not treated with preventive medication. The life expectancy of HIV-infected people is heavily influenced by access to expert medical care.

The majority of opportunistic infections respond to drug treatment when they first appear. AIDS-related cancers are treated with combinations of chemotherapy and radiation therapy. In advanced stages of illness, treatment of multiple infections and cancer may be less successful and complicated by toxic reactions to drugs, especially when several drugs are used in combination.

Research has been aimed at finding drugs that will control HIV. Five antiviral drugs (AZT, ddI, ddC, D4T, 3TC) have been approved. While at least some of these drugs can delay the onset of AIDS in people with HIV and improve the health of people who already have AIDS, the virus eventually becomes resistant to the drugs and the benefits are only temporary.[18] The drugs can also have significant side effects.[19]

Many other drugs are currently being studied. A potent and less toxic class of drugs are called protease inhibitors. Other drugs being investigated include nevirapine, delaviridine, ALX40-4C and SDZ NIM811, antisense oligonucleotides, and gene therapy. Other therapies try to suppress HIV by regulating the function of the immune system. These drugs include IL-2, IL-12, thalidomide, tenidap, and antioxidants.

As new drugs become available, a great deal of research focuses on combining drugs. Some of these combinations have already been shown to have greater effect on the virus and on the immune system than each drug alone, although side effects may also be increased. As of 1995, there are several antivirals to combine but a lack of information available about what is the best combination of antivirals, whether to take drugs in combination or one after another, and when to start drugs. Furthermore, individual responses to antivirals vary widely.

HIV disease is often described as "invariably fatal," but this contradicts the facts. The illness is very serious, and no cure is yet known, but many people have had AIDS for a number of years and are still alive. Some people have been infected with HIV for over ten years and show no signs of illness.[20] As with other serious illnesses such as cancer, increasing medical knowledge and better treatment improve the life expectancy of people with AIDS.

Prevention Is the Best Protection

Development of a vaccine to protect those not yet infected poses formidable problems. The scientific challenge is enormous, and there are ethical problems associated with testing an unproven vaccine for such a dangerous disease. Since these factors make it unlikely that any vaccine will be widely available for years to come, the best way to avoid HIV disease is to understand clearly how it is transmitted and act to prevent transmission from occurring.

TRANSMISSION ROUTES

HIV is known to be transmitted through:

- contact of infected blood, semen, or vaginal and cervical secretions with mucous membranes.
- injection of infected blood or blood products.
- vertical transmission (that is, from infected mother to fetus).

Contact of Sexual Discharges or Blood with Mucous Membranes

The virus cannot pass through undamaged skin. HIV can enter the body through the mucous membranes that line the vagina, rectum, urethra, and possibly the mouth. Damage to a mucous membrane may increase risk of transmission of HIV, but is not necessary.

HIV has consistently been isolated from blood, semen, vaginal and cervical secretions, and breast milk, but only rarely and in low levels from urine, saliva, and tears.[21, 22, 23] Two studies have isolated HIV in pre-ejaculatory fluid.[24, 25] Epidemiological evidence implicates only blood, semen, vaginal and cervical secretions, and breast milk as agents of transmission.[26, 27] Infection through contact of semen, blood, or vaginal or cervical secretions with mucous membranes occurs during anal or vaginal intercourse but only rarely during oral-genital sex. A component of saliva helps inactivate HIV.[28]

Blood into Blood

HIV can be transmitted by infected blood getting directly into the bloodstream through intravenous, intramuscular, or subcutaneous injection. Blood-to-blood transmission occurs in the following ways:

- sharing of unsterilized hypodermic needles and other equipment.
- transfusing of contaminated blood and blood products to hemophiliacs and other blood recipients. Since March 1985 the blood supply has been screened for contaminated blood. The risk of infection from transfusion is now extremely small.

Mother to Fetus

HIV can be transmitted from an infected woman to her fetus during pregnancy and during delivery. This is referred to as vertical transmission. Antiviral therapy (AZT), used at the appropriate time in pregnancy, significantly reduces the risk of transmission from mother to fetus.

NO TRANSMISSION BY CASUAL CONTACT

Every major scientific study has concluded that HIV infection cannot be transmitted by casual contact: "Ordinary standards of personal hygiene that currently prevail are more than adequate for preventing transmission of [HIV] even between persons living within a single household; transmission will not occur as long as one avoids the relatively short list of dangerous sexual and drug-use practices that have been identified."[29] Materials that could theoretically carry the virus in small amounts, such as saliva[30] sprayed in a cough or a sneeze or left on a drinking glass, tears, or urine, have *not* been implicated as the cause of any case of AIDS. The virus is not transmitted by the bites of insects such as ticks or mosquitoes.[31, 32]

HIV Is Fragile

HIV is fragile, much more so than the viruses that cause colds or the flu. It is killed by heat, ordinary soap and water, household bleach solutions, alcohol, hydrogen peroxide, Lysol, and the chlorine used in swimming pools.[33] HIV is not transmitted by contact with inanimate objects.[34]

Families of People with AIDS Remain Healthy Despite Extensive Household Contact

Many studies have been done on transmission patterns within the families of those with HIV infection and AIDS.[35, 36, 37] In these studies no family member or housemate has contracted HIV infection from a person with AIDS other than sexual partners and children born to infected mothers. These people lived together without special precautions, sharing beds, dishes, clothing, toilets, food, toothbrushes, toys, and baby bottles.

Workplace Contact Safe

The Public Health Service states, "AIDS is a blood-borne, sexually transmitted disease that is not spread by casual contact. . . . No known risk of transmission to coworkers, clients, or consumers exists from [HIV] infected workers . . . in offices, schools, factories, or construction sites. . . . Workers known to be infected with [HIV] should not be restricted from work solely based on this finding. Moreover they should not be restricted from using telephones, office equipment, toilets, showers, eating facilities, or water fountains."[38]

2

Observed Patterns of Illness

Scientists at the U.S. Centers for Disease Control (CDC) gather information collected by state and local health departments about each case of AIDS reported and identify the probable route of transmission. CDC statistics are the source for the facts reported below.[1]

In 1979, there were 11 cases of AIDS in the United States. By June 1995, 476,899 cases had been officially reported. AIDS has been reported in all fifty states. AIDS is now the leading cause of death among people twenty-five to forty-four years old.[2]

According to the CDC, by June 1995, there were 470,288 cases in adults and adolescents (age thirteen or over). Routes of transmission were:

- men who have sex with men   52%
- heterosexual contact   8%
- needle sharing by injecting drug users   32%
- transfusion of contaminated blood or blood   2%
  products in the course of medical treatment
  (including treatment for hemophilia)
- not yet assigned a precise mode of transmission   6%

Among the 6,611 cases of AIDS among children younger than thirteen, 90% were caused by vertical transmission (from infected mother to infant during pregnancy, childbirth, or breast feeding).

SEXUAL TRANSMISSION

In 59 to 66% of all adult/adolescent cases of AIDS, the underlying HIV infection was transmitted:

- by sexual activity between men (52% and another possible 7% who may have been infected either through needle sharing or sexual transmission between men).
- By sexual activity between women and men (7%).

Two cases have been attributed to sexual contact between women. In both these cases mucous membranes were exposed to blood as well as to vaginal and cervical secretions.[3]

The percentage of all U.S. cases of AIDS attributed to sexual contact between men and women has increased from 1.2% in 1982 to 8% in 1995. Heterosexual HIV transmission is the most rapidly increasing mode of HIV exposure.[4] In Africa, where more than 70% of all AIDS cases have occurred, sex between men and women has been the most frequent mode of HIV transmission.[5]

Variables Affecting Sexual Transmission

Although sexual transmission of HIV infection in the U.S. has so far occurred most often between men, HIV infection is also sexually transmitted from men to women and from women to men, via vaginal or rectal intercourse. With HIV, a single act of rectal or vaginal intercourse in which semen is deposited in the body may be sufficient for transmission. In the vast majority of cases, however, it appears that repeated exposure to the virus through multiple acts of intercourse has been necessary for transmission to take place.[6]

So far in the United States, many more cases of AIDS have been caused by HIV infection sexually transmitted from men to women than from women to men. This may simply reflect the fact that in this country there are currently more infected men than infected women; or it may also indicate that HIV is more easily transmitted from men to women (as is the case with some other sexually transmitted diseases such as gonorrhea).[7]

In studies of people whose only risk was unprotected sex with HIV-infected partners of the opposite sex, the prevalence of HIV infection ranged from under 10% to as high as 60%.[8] These studies raise the question of why some sexual partners of infected people become infected while others do not. Several factors may affect this[9]:

- Some strains of HIV (such as the HIV subtype commonly seen in Thailand) may be more easily transmissible than others.[10]
- HIV-infected people probably transmit the virus more easily at certain times during the course of infection than at other times; infectiousness probably increases transiently at the time of infection and again as the immune system deteriorates.
- People's ability to transmit the virus may vary depending on the route by which they themselves were infected.
- Concurrent infection with another disease in either partner may make transmission of HIV more likely.[11] Activation of the immune system by illness may make the body more susceptible. Also, mucous membranes in the vagina, rectum, or urethra may be more vulnerable to infection via sexual discharges if sores or other lesions caused by other sexually transmitted diseases are present.
- Type or frequency of sexual exposure may affect susceptibility. For example, the virus may be more easily transmitted through rectal than vaginal intercourse.[12]

Sexually Transmitted AIDS among Non-Needle-Sharing Heterosexuals

By June 1995, an estimated 35,683 cases of AIDS were transmitted by sexual contact between men and women. AIDS transmitted by sexual contact between men and women is already epidemic among the sexual partners of needle-sharers. In some communities heterosexual transmission is also widespread among people who do not share needles. HIV can be transmitted through vaginal intercourse without a condom from male to female and from female to male.

NONSEXUAL TRANSMISSION

Transmission through Needle Sharing

Thirty-two percent of all people with AIDS were probably infected through needle sharing. Needle-sharers probably account for the majority of new infections in the U.S. Some of these may actually have been infected through sexual transmission, particularly the 7% of infected needle-sharers who were men who had had sexual contact with other men. The prevalence of HIV infection among intravenous (IV) drug users varies sharply by geographic region. Over 1.1 million Americans use IV drugs and are therefore potentially at risk for infection if they share needles.[13] A study indicates that 7% of IV drug users become infected with HIV each year.[14] All statistics regarding needle sharing are difficult to verify.

Blood Recipients

Transfusion of blood and blood products in medical treatment was the route of transmission in 3% of cases of AIDS. However, it has been almost eliminated as a source of *new* infections, due to screening of the blood supply.

Hemophiliacs receive blood products called clotting factors that are prepared from many units of donated blood pooled together. Because of this pooling, clotting factors were much more likely to be contaminated with HIV than other blood products, and as a result, hemophiliacs have had a particularly high rate of infection. Treatment with heat and chemicals has eliminated clotting factors as sources of new infections.[15]

Approximately 20 million patients received blood transfusions from 1980 through 1985, when screening of the blood supply for HIV began. There were 751 new cases of HIV attributable to transfusion reported in 1994. Nearly all of these cases were due to transfusions received before 1985. Blood products that are *known* to have transmitted HIV are whole blood, blood cellular components, plasma, and clotting factors. Blood products that are not known to have ever transmitted HIV are immunoglobulin, albumin, plasma protein fraction, and hepatitis B vaccine.

Vertical Transmission

Vertical transmission is the term used to describe HIV transmission from mother to infant. It is also sometimes referred to as perinatal transmission. HIV infection can be transmitted from mother to fetus during pregnancy, to the infant during delivery, or through infected breast milk.[16] The mother need not have any symptoms; she need only be HIV-infected. Of the 6,611 children with AIDS, 90% have been infected by an HIV-infected mother. It is estimated that from 30 to 50% of infections occur during pregnancy (probably mostly during later stages of pregnancy), and 50 to 60% occur during labor and delivery.[17, 18, 19] A small number of cases of transmission through HIV-infected human breast milk have been reported in the United States. It is recommended that HIV-infected women in the United States (and other areas where safe alternatives to breast-feeding exist) not breast-feed their infants.[20, 21]

The pregnancy of an infected woman has a significant chance of resulting in a baby born with HIV infection:

studies quote probabilities from 15 to 40%.[22, 23, 24] At present, the majority of children with AIDS (people under the age of thirteen) had mothers who were injecting-drug users or were sex partners of injecting-drug users.[25]

Several strategies are being developed to reduce the risk of vertical transmission. An important study has indicated that appropriate use of the antiviral drug AZT reduced the risk of mother–infant transmission by two-thirds.[26] In this study, women who were mildly asymptomatic were given AZT during pregnancy and labor, and their infants were given AZT for the first six weeks of life. Other promising strategies for reducing mother–infant transmission are being studied.

Fertility of women does not appear to be affected by HIV infection. There is currently no scientific agreement on whether a pregnancy accelerates the course of HIV disease in an HIV-infected woman.

Medical Personnel

Tens of thousands of health care workers treat AIDS patients every day. Health care workers include doctors, nurses, surgeons, dentists, and others. Many health care workers have either accidentally stuck themselves with needles used to treat AIDS patients or been splashed with blood or other body fluids of patients. The risk of becoming infected through a skin puncture with blood *known* to be infected is estimated at about one in three hundred.[27] As of June 1995, there were forty-six documented reports of health care workers in the United States having been infected through their work, thirty-seven through skin punctures. Eighteen laboratory technicians have been infected, sixteen nurses, six physicians, and no surgeons or dentists.[28] Health care workers can greatly reduce their risk of infection via exposure to blood by adhering strictly and uniformly to infection-control procedures recommended by the CDC.[29]

There is only one instance reported of a health care

worker transmitting the virus to patients. A dentist in Florida apparently infected six of his patients. The circumstances surrounding this are not entirely clear. This is, so far, a unique situation.[30]

Few with Undetermined Risk

Six percent of all cases of AIDS fall into a transmission category that the CDC labels as "other/risk not reported or identified." As of June 1995, 29,652 people were reported in this category. Over 19,000 are people whose cases have not yet been completely investigated by the CDC. Almost 6,000 could not be further investigated, due to death, inability to follow up, or declining interview. Only 827 cases that have been completely investigated could not be reclassified into a known exposure category on the basis of elicited information.[31]

SOME DEMOGRAPHIC FACTS

Gay Men and AIDS

AIDS is now the leading cause of death among men between twenty-five and forty-four years of age. In 1995 alone more young Americans will die from AIDS than perished in the entire decade of the Vietnam War, and the majority of them will be gay. Unfortunately, HIV infection had already spread widely among gay men before AIDS was recognized and modes of transmission were understood. The gay community's extraordinary efforts in major urban centers toward risk reduction, public health education, and the support and care of people with AIDS have set an example for community response to the epidemic.

Risk reduction for HIV infection has been widely adopted in the gay community. A study done in San Francisco indicated that high-risk behavior among the gay men studied had decreased 90% between 1978 and 1985.[32] However, recent information is more discouraging. From

July 1994 to June 1995, the percentage of cases transmitted by sex between men was 43% of the total, but in men from ages twenty to twenty-four, 60% of cases were transmitted by sex between men.[33] In a study of gay and bisexual San Francisco men, ages seventeen to twenty-two, about one-third of the participants reported unprotected anal intercourse in the last six months.[34] A similar study of young gay men in New York found even higher rates of anal intercourse without condoms.[35] These figures indicate a pressing need for ongoing AIDS education in the gay community, especially among young people. New strategies must be developed that take into account the difficulty of maintaining risk reduction over a long time and the psychological effects of the epidemic on non-HIV-infected gay men.

Outside major urban areas, risk-reduction education for gay men remains inadequate. Nationwide, societal hostility to gay men combines with disapproval of sexual activity to hinder safe-sex educational efforts. Stigmatization deprives closeted men of the supportive consensus for risk reduction that has developed among openly gay Americans.

Women with AIDS

Women account for over 13% of all adult/adolescent cases of AIDS reported in this country so far. The proportion of cases among women has steadily increased in the last ten years. From July 1994 to June 1995, women represented 18% of new adult/adolescent AIDS cases. The vast majority of women with AIDS are of reproductive age: 87% are between the ages of thirteen and forty-nine. There were 64,822 women with AIDS as of June 1995. Forty-seven percent of these women were infected by needle sharing. Thirty-six percent were infected through heterosexual contact, more than half of which were infected by sex with an injecting-drug user.[36]

There is an emerging epidemic of HIV among young women of color in the Southeast and in New York City associated with cocaine crack use and trading sex for drugs or money.

In the United States, women with AIDS have a higher rate of mortality than men with AIDS. This may reflect a difference in access to care and socioeconomic factors such as poverty, homelessness, substance abuse, and domestic violence rather than a biological difference.[37]

Children with AIDS

Children under thirteen years of age account for about 1.5% of all cases of AIDS in the United States. Eighty-nine percent of these children were infected by their mothers before or at birth, and another 10% were infected through contaminated blood or blood products.

Hemophiliacs and AIDS

An estimated 15,000 to 20,000 Americans have either hemophilia A or hemophilia B. From 22 to 42% of hemophiliacs are HIV-infected. The tragically high prevalence of infection among hemophiliacs is due to the fact that clotting factor is prepared from blood pooled from a large number of donors. Before screening of donated blood was instituted in March 1985, clotting factor was likely to be contaminated with HIV. Heat treatment of U.S.-manufactured clotting-factor concentrates has eliminated this risk of infection for those hemophiliacs who remain uninfected and those born since 1985.[38]

Ethnicity and AIDS

Of the reported cases of people with AIDS in the United States as of June 1995, 48% were white, 33% were African-American, and 17% were Hispanic. African-American and Hispanic people represent only 12% and 6%, respectively, of the U.S. population and are therefore overrepresented among people with AIDS. Most women with AIDS were African-American (55%) or Hispanic (20%). In 1994, the rate (number of cases per 100,000 people) of AIDS cases reported was six times higher among African-Americans than whites and three times higher among Hispanics than whites. Among children with AIDS, 56% are African-American.

Individuals are not at higher risk for AIDS because of their race or ethnicity. The disproportion of AIDS among African-American and Hispanic people occurs in cases that were transmitted by needle sharing. The high incidence of IV drug use and needle sharing in some African-American and Hispanic communities is due to the combined impact of underlying social and economic factors including poverty, racism, unequal schooling, and unequal opportunity for employment. Further, African-American and Hispanic communities are concentrated in the large urban areas, which have a high incidence of HIV infection.

The spread of HIV infection among African-American and Hispanic needle-sharers has continued essentially unchecked: AIDS education and prevention has largely been targeted toward a white, middle-class population and has not adequately addressed the issues relevant to needle-sharers, who generally have much poorer access to information and medical services. There is a severe shortage of treatment facilities for people who wish to stop using drugs.

White people with AIDS have a life expectancy from time of diagnosis that is two to three times longer than that for African-American people with AIDS. This is probably due to social factors (poor health care, drug-related problems, nutritional status) rather than to biological differences.

AIDS INTERNATIONALLY

As of 1995, there were estimated to be 4.5 million cases of AIDS worldwide and 16 to 19.5 million cases of HIV infection.[39] According to the World Health Organization

(WHO) the estimated distribution of HIV infection from the late 1970s to mid-1994 is as follows[40]:

• Sub-Saharan Africa	10 million +
• South and Southeast Asia	2.5 million +
• Latin America and the Caribbean	2 million
• North America	1 million +
• Western Europe	500,000 +
• North Africa and the Middle East	100,000
• Eastern Europe and Central Asia	50,000 +
• East Asia and the Pacific	50,000
• Australia	25,000 +

It is estimated that sub-Saharan Africa has suffered 64% of the total cases of HIV infection worldwide and that one in forty men and women in sub-Saharan Africa are currently infected. Prevention programs are tragically limited, and medical treatment that might reduce suffering and limit mother–infant transmission is usually not available.

PROJECTIONS FOR THE FUTURE

Epidemiologists and social scientists have developed a number of models for predicting the incidence of AIDS in the future. These figures are, of course, only estimates. Following are some predictions regarding AIDS in the United States and internationally:

• The World Health Organization has projected that 42 million people will be HIV-infected in the year 2000.[41]
• One expert postulated a "moderate" estimate of 5,861,000 cases of HIV infection in the United States by 2002.[42]
• Another scientist estimates a cumulative total of 7 million people in the United States infected by 2009.[43]

3

Prevention

Learn to distinguish situations in which there is a real possibility of HIV transmission from situations with little or no risk of transmission. In common, everyday nonsexual activities you do not need to take special precautions. In certain sexual activities and in use of injected drugs, you need to take steps to reduce the risk of transmission of HIV.

NO DANGER FROM CASUAL CONTACT

There is no danger of contracting HIV infection through casual contact. However, observe routine and reasonable precautions against accidental contact with blood, semen, or vaginal secretions. Wash hands or skin with soap and water. Clean surfaces where blood or semen have been spilled with soap and water or a mild disinfectant solution such as 10% household bleach. Do not share toothbrushes, razors, tweezers, or other instruments that may carry fresh blood. These precautions provide protection against many common illnesses.

Service Occupations No Hazard
The U.S. Public Health Service has made a series of recommendations regarding HIV infection in the workplace.

These recommendations explicitly say that transmission of HIV is unlikely even in work settings in which close nonsexual person-to-person contact occurs. The occupations considered fall into three categories:

- Food service workers including cooks, waiters, bartenders, and airline attendants.
- Personal-service workers including hairdressers, barbers, cosmetologists, and manicurists.
- Health care workers including nurses, doctors, dentists, optometrists, lab technicians, and emergency medical technicians.

The Public Health Service (PHS) states: "All laboratory and epidemiological evidence indicates that blood-borne and sexually transmitted infections are not transmitted during the preparation or serving of food or beverages, and no instances of [HIV] transmission have been documented in this setting."[1]

The PHS found no evidence of transmission of HIV from personal-service workers to clients or vice versa.

Health care workers known to be infected with HIV need not be restricted from work unless they have evidence of other infection or illness for which any health care worker would be restricted. Since blood is often present during medical procedures and is a source of transmission of HIV, the PHS has outlined routine hygiene procedures to prevent the transmission of HIV in a health care setting.[2]

No Risk of Casual Transmission from Child to Child

Since the start of the AIDS epidemic, there has been public and media concern about the possibility that young children with AIDS might somehow infect their schoolmates in ordinary day-to-day interactions. In some cases, fearful parents have harassed sick children and attempted to have them removed from school. Such fear is not warranted by scientific evidence. No case of AIDS has been transmitted in a school or day-care setting.

Due to sexual activity and intravenous drug use, adolescents face a much greater risk for becoming HIV-infected than younger children.

Blood Transfusion Much Safer since 1985

People who were transfused with many units of blood in the few years prior to late spring 1985 are at increased risk of being HIV-infected, especially if these transfusions occurred in areas with a high incidence of HIV infection (New York, San Francisco, and Los Angeles). Such people are unlikely to be infected but should seek counseling about HIV-antibody testing.[3]

Giving Blood Has Always Been Safe

There is absolutely no risk of becoming infected with HIV from donating blood, and there never has been, since the needles used to draw blood are sterile-packaged and are never reused. If you are at risk for being HIV-infected and you are pressured into participating in a blood donation drive, be sure to indicate on the form provided that you wish to donate your blood for *research purposes only*. This option is standard and is provided by blood banks to protect your privacy while helping you avoid any embarrassment associated with refusing to donate blood.

AVOID NEEDLE SHARING

You face high risk for HIV infection if you share needles, whether to inject or "skin-pop" heroin, cocaine, speed, or any other drug. Also, if you are already infected, drugs themselves may increase the chance that your infection will make you ill. HIV-infected injecting-drug users who continue to shoot drugs have a worse course of illness than those who stop using needles.[4]

If you continue to inject drugs, it is crucially important that you do not share IV drug equipment ("works," "gimmicks," "sets"), including syringes, rubber bulbs, needles ("points"), "cookers," or cotton. If you buy new works, clean them *before* using them. If you share works, clean them before you or the next person uses them. Blood may be in your works even if you can't see it. Clean your works either with rubbing alcohol (available in drugstores), a household bleach solution (three tablespoons of bleach in a cup of water), or boiling water. To clean your works:

- Pour the alcohol, bleach solution, or boiling water into a clean glass.
- Pull liquid up into the syringe, shake well, then squirt the liquid out again. Repeat this several times.
- Take your works apart, separating the plunger and needle from the syringe.
- Let them soak in the alcohol, bleach solution, or boiling water for ten to fifteen minutes.
- Rinse the parts of your works well under running tap water.
- Put your works back together. Pull clean water up into the syringe, then squirt it out again. Repeat a few times.

If you can't wait, use the bleach solution, skip the soaking step, and be sure to rinse thoroughly with water.

Remember, no matter how you got infected, you can still pass it on through sex.

An estimated 1.2 million Americans use IV drugs regularly. The proportion of IV drug users in treatment programs who have been found to be HIV infected varies from 0% in Cheyenne, Wyoming, to 61% in New York City.[5] Existing treatment programs can accommodate only one in every twelve IV drug users. In New York City, the average waiting period to get into a methadone maintenance program is one to three months. The waiting period to get into a drug-free program where addicts are kept "clean" of all drugs is up to six months.[6]

Studies show that education about AIDS and clean needles leads IV drug users not only to adopt HIV-safer injection techniques, but to seek treatment for their drug problem. A leading medical and public-health authority on IV drug abuse offers the following recommendations[7]:

- Large-scale expansion of drug-abuse treatment programs.
- Face-to-face health-promotion activities conducted by former IV drug users.
- More teaching of needle-cleaning methods and/or distribution of sterile needles.
- Support of self-help groups of IV drug users who work to legitimize safe sex and the refusal to share needles.

The National Academy of Sciences has also recommended experimenting with legalization of the sale and possession of sterile disposable needles and syringes as a public-health measure to reduce HIV transmission through needle sharing.[8]

HAVE SEX SAFELY

It is never too late to begin protecting yourself against HIV. Even if you have reason to believe you have already been infected, it is always to your benefit to follow sexual risk-reduction guidelines since repeat exposure to HIV or exposure to other sexually transmitted infections may help to trigger illness. Follow the risk-reduction guidelines below in any future sexual encounter.

Sexual Risk-Reduction Guidelines

Safer sex in one sentence: use a condom for every episode of intercourse, from start to finish, whether vaginal or rectal.

More detailed risk-reduction guidelines divide common

sexual behaviors into three categories of risk for transmitting HIV: high-risk, lower-risk, and no-risk. Behaviors in the high-risk category generally involve contact of blood or semen with a mucous membrane. Mucous membranes include the linings of the rectum, vagina, mouth, and urethra (the tube through which urine is passed). Contact of blood or semen with a mucous membrane has a *high risk* of transmitting HIV if one partner is infected—avoid sexual activities involving such contact.

If there is no contact between one partner's bodily fluids and the other partner's mucous membranes, there is *no risk* of infection—transmission of HIV cannot occur. No-risk sexual activities are therefore completely safe even if one or both partners is infected.

The situation is less clear-cut in the case of the lower-risk category. Behaviors in this category involve some risk of mucous membrane contact with bodily fluids other than blood and semen. These fluids occasionally contain HIV, but at a low concentration that makes infection much less likely. Saliva is almost certainly safe, and it is unlikely that the virus enters the body through the mucous membranes of the mouth.[9] It is impossible to prove that lower-risk behaviors will never transmit the virus, but these behaviors are much less dangerous than those in the high-risk category. In cases where one or both sexual partners may be carrying the virus, the partners should carefully discuss exactly which lower-risk activities are acceptable to both of them.

The greater the chance that your partner is infected, the greater the risk of infection through sex. Men who have had unprotected sex with other men and people who have shared needles for IV drug use are statistically at greatest risk of being infected, but most sexually active people are at some risk for HIV infection.

In the following pages, common sexual activities are listed with a brief explanation of why they are considered to be high-risk, lower-risk, or no-risk.

High-Risk Activities

High-risk activities have a high probability of transmitting HIV infection, especially if either partner is a man who has had unprotected sex with other men or is a man or woman who has shared needles. If you have sex and you do not explicitly know that both you and your partner are uninfected, avoid high-risk sexual activities.

Vaginal or Rectal Intercourse without a Condom

If ejaculation (coming) occurs while the penis is inside the vagina or rectum, the mucous lining of the vagina or rectum is exposed to semen, which may contain a high level of HIV. Use adequate lubricant to reduce abrasion or other damage to the vagina or rectum; infection can happen even if no abrasion occurs. Using a condom to contain the semen lowers the risk of infection considerably, but condoms may break or leak. If ejaculation occurs and semen escapes, there is a risk of infection. For this reason, intercourse with a condom is safer if the penis is withdrawn before ejaculation.

Being the receptive partner during unprotected rectal or vaginal intercourse has been highly associated with contracting HIV infection. Being the insertive partner during unprotected vaginal or rectal intercourse can also lead to HIV infection, probably via exposure to secretions or menstrual blood in the vagina, or to blood in the rectum. During intercourse, the insertive partner's urethral lining may be exposed to infected fluid that enters through the opening in the tip of the penis.

Fellatio (Sucking, Blow Job) with Ejaculation into Partner's Mouth

Fellatio is stimulation of the penis with the mouth. There appears to be virtually no danger to the insertive partner (the person putting his penis in the other person's mouth). There is controversy about the level of safety of fellatio to the receptive partner (the person in whose mouth the penis is placed). It is a reasonable conclusion based on currently available information that transmission to the receptive partner by fellatio can occur, but is probably quite rare.

There are some documented cases of infection occurring from fellatio.[10] It appears that HIV was transmitted by ejaculation of semen (coming) into the partner's mouth. However, some of the case reports do not indicate whether ejaculation occurred in the mouth.

The risk of fellatio to the receptive partner is probably considerably lower if the penis is withdrawn before ejaculation. See the section on fellatio that follows under "Lower-Risk Activities." The risk of fellatio is low if the insertive partner wears a condom.

Cunnilingus (Oral Sex) during Menstruation

Cunnilingus is stimulation of a woman's genitals with the lips and tongue. Cunnilingus during menstruation is high-risk for the partner performing cunnilingus because there may be a high concentration of virus in menstrual blood. See the section on cunnilingus that follows under "Lower-Risk Activities."

Oral-Anal Contact (Rimming)

Oral-anal contact is stimulation of the anus with the lips and tongue. It is high-risk because blood that may be present in the rectum may contact the lining of the mouth. The risk is for the partner performing the oral-anal contact. This is not a likely route of transmission of HIV but is likely to transmit intestinal parasites, which can produce serious medical problems and exacerbate an existing HIV infection.

Lower-Risk Activities

These activities have only a small chance of transmitting HIV infection. When having sex with a man who has had unprotected sex with other men or with people who have shared needles, discuss which, if any, lower-risk sexual activities you are willing to perform.

Vaginal and Rectal Intercourse with Condoms and without Ejaculation Inside Partner's Body

Condoms are an effective barrier to virus transmission.[11] Using a condom lowers the risk of infection considerably. However, condoms may break or leak. If ejaculation occurs and semen escapes, there is a risk of infection. Be sure to use condoms correctly (see the section below on condoms). Intercourse with a condom is much safer if the penis is withdrawn before ejaculation.

Fellatio without Ejaculation into Partner's Mouth

The risk of transmission from fellatio is thought to be much lower than the risk of unprotected intercourse. However, since semen may contain a relatively high concentration of virus, it is wisest to avoid contact of semen with the lining of the mouth.[12] Studies attempting to assess the relative danger of oral sex for HIV transmission have had conflicting results, and it is currently not possible to quantify the risk of oral sex.[13, 14, 15]

If fellatio is not continued to ejaculation, the mucous membranes of the mouth are not exposed to semen. This probably lowers the risk of fellatio significantly. Two small studies have shown that pre-ejaculatory fluid ("pre-cum") contains some virus. (Pre-ejaculatory fluid is a viscous, clear fluid that is secreted from the penis sometime prior to the ejaculation of semen itself.) The risk is further reduced if the head of the penis is never placed in the mouth or if a condom is worn. Kissing or licking the shaft of the penis is safe.

Cunnilingus Not during Menstruation

If menstruation is not occurring, the mucous membranes of the mouth are not exposed to blood. This lowers the risk of infection during cunnilingus considerably. However, vaginal and cervical secretions sometimes contain a low concentration of virus. The small risk associated with cunnilingus is lowered still further if an effective barrier such as a square of latex or plastic wrap (called an oral dam) is used to separate the genitals from the partner's lips and tongue.

Oral-Anal Contact (Rimming) with a Barrier

The risk associated with oral-anal contact is made much lower if an effective barrier is used to keep the lips and tongue from contacting the partner's anus.

Deep Kissing (French Kissing, Tongue Kissing)

Studies have indicated that the virus is sometimes present in saliva, but only at very low levels. There is no evidence that exchange of saliva transmits the virus, even in prolonged deep kissing. No cases of AIDS transmitted by kissing alone have been reported.

No-Risk Activities

Mutual Masturbation, Rubbing Bodies, and Kissing Skin Are Examples

If your partner's bodily fluids do not contact your mucous membranes, you cannot be infected with HIV.

Condom Information

Condoms can prevent the transmission of HIV and also provide protection against diseases such as gonorrhea, chlamydial infections, syphilis, and herpes.[16, 17] Other methods of birth control, such as using a diaphragm with spermicide, do not provide adequate protection against the transmission of HIV infection and other sexually transmitted diseases. Condoms can be bought at drugstores (no prescription is needed).

Use Condoms Correctly

- Condoms are latex, polyurethane, or animal-membrane sheaths that fit over the erect penis and act as a barrier to prevent semen or pre-cum from escaping while the penis is inside the vagina or rectum. Use only latex or polyurethane condoms. Do not use animal-membrane condoms; they contain pores through which HIV can pass.[18] Polyurethane condoms became available in 1995. While there is less data regarding their safety in practice (reducing transmission of STDs and pregnancy), there is evidence that the material they are made of is even less porous than latex. Consequently, they should prove to be at least as safe as latex condoms. The advantages of polyurethane condoms are that they can be used with oil-based lubricants (such as Vaseline and baby oil), they are thinner than latex condoms, and they transmit heat better. This means that polyurethane condoms will feel more "natural" to some people. The disadvantage of polyurethane condoms is that they will probably be more expensive. They may be particularly useful to the small group of people who are allergic to latex.
- Do not use condoms that are ribbed or textured to increase stimulation since these condoms may cause damage to genital tissues that, while unnoticeable, may make infection more likely.
- Store condoms in a cool, dry place, out of direct sunlight. Condoms kept in wallets may become damaged over time. Condoms are considered to be good for two years after their date of manufacture, which is sometimes printed on the package.
- The condom should be put on the penis after it is erect, not before. Put on the condom before the penis comes in contact with the genitals or with the anus.

- Condoms come packaged either rolled-up or loose. If the condom is rolled up, determine which side is the inside of the condom, place that side against the tip of the penis, and roll the rest of the condom down to the base. The condom should fit snugly so that it does not slip off during intercourse. If the condom is packaged unrolled, draw it over the penis like a glove.

- When putting on a condom, pinch about one-half inch of the condom's tip to leave a small air-free space—this will help keep semen from bursting the condom upon ejaculation. If the penis is uncircumcised, retract the foreskin before putting on the condom.

- If intercourse is continued to ejaculation, the penis should be withdrawn promptly afterward. Since condoms may break or leak, ejaculation inside the body presents a risk of infection.

- In any case, the condom-covered penis should be withdrawn from the vagina or rectum before the penis becomes soft. During withdrawal, hold the rim of the condom firmly against the penis so that the condom cannot slip off and no semen can escape.

- Do not reuse condoms.

- In 1994, so-called female condoms became commercially available. Studies indicate that female condoms are effective in preventing transmission of HIV.[19, 20] The technical name of these devices is lubricated polyurethane bags. These are polyurethane devices that are inserted into the vagina or rectum in order to create a protective barrier and prevent contact of semen with the mucous membrane of the vagina or rectum. The advantages of these condoms is that the receptive partner has more control over their use and that these condoms can be inserted many hours before sex. Their disadvantage is that they are expensive and some people find them uncomfortable or aesthetically displeasing.[21]

Lubricants Should Be Water Based

Lubrication is important to avoid tearing the condom or abrading body tissue. With latex condoms always use a water-based lubricant such as K-Y jelly, ForPlay, or Probe; never use oil-based lubricants such as hand lotion, Vaseline, Crisco, baby oil, vegetable oil, mineral oil, suntan lotion, Albolene, Elbow Grease, Lube, or Shaft, since these may damage the latex of the condom. Oil-based lubricants can be used with polyurethane condoms. Put a drop of lubricant inside the tip of the condom before it is put on the penis. Too much lubricant inside the condom may cause it to slip off during intercourse. Use a generous amount of lubricant on the outside of the condom.

Nonoxynol-9 Provides Extra Protection

A spermicide called nonoxynol-9 is found in some contraceptive jellies and creams as well as in many lubricants. Preparations that contain at least 5% nonoxynol-9 provide extra protection when used with condoms since this concentration has been shown to kill HIV.[22] A water- and glycerin-based lubricant called ForPlay™ will not weaken or damage the latex of condoms and contains 5% nonoxynol-9. Some brands of condoms now come coated inside and out with a 5% nonoxynol-9 lubricant. One such brand is *LifeStyles Extra-Strength™ Condoms with Nonoxynol-9.* A number of contraceptive creams, jellies, and foams contain nonoxynol-9, but not all contain enough. A small number of people are allergic to nonoxynol-9. Also, most products intended as spermicides dry out quickly and so do not make good lubricants.

Additional Guidelines

Sex toys (dildos, vibrators, etc.) should not be shared. Clean sex toys thoroughly with soap and water.

Wash the genitals with soap and water after sex. Douching or enemas immediately before or after sex do not help protect you against infection and may even increase the risk of infection by damaging natural protective barriers of the vagina or rectum.[23] Do not put chemicals not intended for internal use into your vagina or rectum.

Urine may contain the virus. Do not allow urine to enter the mouth or come in contact with open cuts on the body.

If you have sores or abrasions on your genitals, anus, or mouth, avoid activity that brings these into contact with your sexual partners. Also, if you have another sexually transmitted disease, have only no-risk sex until you are healthy. The presence of any one of a variety of sexually transmitted diseases may increase the risk of transmission of HIV infection.[24]

If a partner's semen accidentally gets inside your vagina or rectum, you may use spermicide (possibly containing nonoxynol-9) to reduce the risk of infection. If semen gets in your mouth, spit it out and gargle with fresh mouthwash, toothpaste, or even soap and water if nothing else is available.

Adapting to Risk Reduction

Simply limiting the number of your sexual partners is not sufficient precaution against HIV infection. Two related misconceptions date from the early stages of the epidemic in this country: first, that having had many sexual partners somehow in and of itself causes AIDS; and second, that if you have had a small number of sexual partners, you are not at risk for AIDS.

Even if you have only one sexual partner, that person may be infected. Repeated unsafe sexual contact with one infected partner exposes you to a high risk of becoming infected yourself.

The more partners you have, the greater the odds are that at least one of your partners will be infected. However, if you consistently avoid all high-risk sexual activity with all your partners, the extra risk associated with multiple sexual partners becomes much less significant.

Talk about Safe Sex with Your Partners

Men who have had unprotected sex with other men or those of either sex who have shared needles for IV drug use have an increased risk of being infected with HIV. A partner who does not fit either of these descriptions has lower but not zero risk. Bring up the subject of risk reduction with potential sexual partners. Information about level of risk is useful only to the extent that you trust your partner's honesty about this subject. If you cannot talk to your partners frankly, then, for purposes of deciding about safe sex, you should act as if your partners were infected.

Intuition Is an Unreliable Guide

You cannot tell whether a sexual partner is infected from appearance or social behavior. If you do not know a partner well, then you cannot know the level of risk and you should avoid all high-risk sexual activities.

Strike a Balance

Some people become so afraid of HIV infection that they give up sex, or alternate abstinence with occasional impulsive episodes of high-risk sex. Others deny that the epidemic has any chance of affecting them and continue high-risk sexual behavior without an appropriate level of concern. Extremes of behavior (anxious and fragile abstinence, unconcerned high-risk sex) may lead to a high risk of infection. A middle course usually represents a better strategy. You need not give up your sex life nor should you expose yourself to high-risk sexual activity. Many people have been practicing risk-reduction for several years now. They report that although it was sometimes difficult at the beginning, they are now able to enjoy sex that is both safe and satisfying.

Planning for Risk Reduction

Learn how to come to an agreement with your partner about the sexual activity you will have together. Think through the issues in advance. This will help you avoid impulsive decisions and give a clear and consistent message to your partner. Have condoms available if you plan to have intercourse. Women hesitant to purchase and carry condoms should be aware that women now buy half of all condoms sold. The use of alcohol or other recreational drugs often impairs judgment; do not make decisions about sexual activity while you are intoxicated.

Try to talk about risk reduction with your partners before sexual excitement interferes. Many have found that prospective partners interpret raising the subject of risk reduction well before sex as a sign of intelligence and prudence. Others prefer to wait until they are actually involved in explicit sexual activity; follow this course of action only if you can stick to your decisions about risk reduction and if you know that your partner will respect your wishes.

Ask yourself the following questions:

- Have you been practicing risk reduction *consistently*?
- If not, what issues or circumstances interfere?
- How can you resolve these issues or avoid these circumstances?

If you are having difficulty avoiding high-risk sex, get help and support from an AIDS organization in your community. Many such organizations run "safe sex workshops" designed to help with this problem.

Men who have sex with both women and men face difficult issues regarding risk reduction. Ideally, discuss your sexual history with all your partners, both male and female, so that they may make informed decisions about risk reduction. Practice risk reduction with both women and men to avoid infecting yourself or others.

Frank discussion of risk reduction may be difficult for men who have not told their female partners about sexual relations with other men. If your sexual contact with men has never involved the exchange of bodily fluids, you pose no special risk to your female partners. However, if there is a chance that you may already be infected, then you must practice risk reduction with your female as well as your male partners: at a minimum, use condoms. If there is a chance you may be infected and you cannot tell your female partners, seek counseling from an AIDS organization in your community.

4

HIV Antibody Testing

The HIV antibody test is a blood test that, if properly used, can tell you whether you have been infected with HIV. Medical opinion now strongly recommends that if you are at some risk of being HIV-infected, you should be anonymously tested for HIV antibodies so that if you are infected, you can benefit from recent dramatic advances in medical care. People infected with HIV can now get special medical care *before* the development of any noticeable symptoms—care that has been shown to delay AIDS and extend life.

Since HIV may be transmitted mother-to-fetus, you should also be tested if you are thinking of having a child and either you or your partner has any risk of infection (including having had multiple sexual partners of the opposite sex).

The test indicates whether your blood contains antibodies to HIV. Antibodies are proteins manufactured by your immune system that signal the presence—at some prior time or now—of unwanted foreign material such as bacteria or viruses that may have entered your body. Each antibody is specific to a particular kind of foreign material.

A "positive" HIV antibody test result means antibodies to this virus were detected. A "negative" result means antibodies to this virus were not detected. If the test detects antibodies to HIV, it means that you have at some point been infected by HIV and you must consider yourself capable of transmitting the virus. In contrast to many other infections, the presence of antibodies to HIV does not mean that you have successfully fought off infection.

HIV antibody testing is often incorrectly referred to as the "AIDS" test. Having a positive antibody test result does not mean you have AIDS now; however, a positive result *does* mean that you face a significant chance of dangerous illness in the future if you do not receive treatment.

Because of possible discrimination, you should be tested only under conditions of guaranteed anonymity. Speak to a trained counselor at a service specifically set up to do HIV antibody test counseling. Your doctor is not necessarily trained to understand the social and legal issues surrounding the HIV antibody test.

PRECONDITIONS FOR SAFE AND MEANINGFUL TESTING

Testing is only safe, meaningful, and productive if certain preconditions are fulfilled. Before being tested you must thoroughly understand the facts of testing. If infected, you should be under the care of an expert physician, even if you have no symptoms. Obtaining this specialized medical care requires thought and planning; antibody testing without expert medical care will do nothing to protect your health.

Delay of Months before Antibodies May Be Detectable

The body does not manufacture HIV antibodies immediately after infection. Most people develop measurable levels of antibodies in the blood within a few weeks after infection with HIV, but some people may take longer before their blood tests positive. Six months is considered a reasonable time to wait after the last possible time of infection before being tested. Therefore, HIV antibody testing is only meaningful if enough time has passed since the last possible exposure to the virus. If not enough time has passed, the antibody test result may be negative despite the fact that the virus itself is present. Because the delay in antibody formation—sometimes called the window period—might defeat screening of the blood supply in a small number of cases, those at risk for being HIV-infected should not donate blood.[1, 2]

Accurate Testing May Require a Sequence of Tests

HIV antibody testing provides accurate information only if it is done properly. Under certain circumstances a single blood specimen may be tested with a sequence of different tests. A very sensitive test called the EIA test (enzyme immunoassay, formerly referred to as the ELISA test) is used first. If the blood sample is negative on the EIA test, then the laboratory will report a negative result. If the first EIA is positive, the laboratory should repeat the EIA test. If repeated EIA tests are positive, a separate confirmatory test (usually Western blot analysis) is performed on the same blood specimen. If the Western blot analysis is positive, the laboratory will report a positive result.

Some Western blot analysis results cannot be conclusively determined to be either positive or negative. Such results are reported by the laboratory as "inconclusive" or "indeterminate." If your test is indeterminate, consult with your testing counselor. Generally, you should wait four weeks and then repeat the test. If your second test is also indeterminate, you should wait another four weeks and then be tested a third time; this time, in addition to the EIA and a confirming test, the laboratory should use additional tests such as immunofluorescent assay or DNA amplification via polymerase chain reaction (PCR).[3, 4, 5]

False Positives Do Occur

When performed by a good laboratory, the EIA–Western blot testing sequence is extremely accurate. However, the quality of laboratories varies, and technical errors could cause an uninfected person to be falsely identified as infected: a "false positive" result. When screening populations in which the incidence of HIV infection is very *low*, such errors may mean that a substantial proportion of the positive results reported by the test sequence may be false.[6] If your test result is positive and your risk was low, repeat testing with a new blood specimen.

Positive Result Indicates Opportunity for Treatment

If you have a positive HIV antibody test result (also known as being antibody-positive or seropositive), then you must assume you are infected and could possibly infect others through sexual contact, needle sharing, or childbearing. A positive HIV antibody test result indicates infection with HIV but provides no information about the current degree of illness or risk for opportunistic infections. Without treatment, 78 to 100% of HIV-infected people will develop AIDS within fifteen years of infection.[7, 8] Therefore, if you are HIV-positive, you should be seen by a physician with expertise on HIV infection so that you can obtain treatment to slow or stop progression toward AIDS. See the next chapter for more information.

Negative Result Does Not Indicate Immunity

If you have a negative HIV antibody test result (also known as being antibody-negative or seronegative) and the test was performed at least six months after the last possible exposure to HIV, then your result indicates that you have not been infected with the virus, you cannot infect others, and you have no current risk of developing HIV illness. All people should be aware that a negative test result does not mean that you are immune to possible infection in the future.

ANONYMOUS TESTING IS AVAILABLE

In order to protect yourself from possible discrimination (see below) you should be tested anonymously. HIV antibody testing is anonymous only if those doing the testing never know your real name, address, or any other identifying information. In anonymous testing you are assigned a code that identifies your blood specimen without revealing your identity.

OTHER ADVICE ABOUT HIV ANTIBODY TESTING

Prepare for Psychological Stress

A positive antibody test result will almost certainly cause you psychological distress. Living with this stress has been painful and damaging for many people, according to evidence gathered by psychologists. In some cases this stress has led to serious psychological problems including severe anxiety and depression. It is best to discuss your situation with a trained AIDS counselor both before you are tested and after you receive your results. Government-sponsored anonymous test sites generally provide counseling. Counseling tends to be inadequate in private doctors' offices. Since testing positive leads to great psychological stress, you should get additional support after such a test result, either informally through friends, through HIV support groups, or through professional counseling. It may be helpful to locate sources of such support before being tested.

Testing Not Generally Useful for Risk Reduction

Some have argued that HIV antibody testing will increase motivation to adopt risk-reduction behavior. No evidence supports this assertion. Expert opinion suggests that the best route to productive behavior change is through education, support, and counseling, not antibody testing.

Some people seek testing in the hope that they will

be antibody-negative and so will be able to discontinue practicing risk reduction. Having high-risk sex is prudent only if you and your partner have both tested antibody-negative twice (where the first and second tests were performed at least six months apart) and have had no other sexual partners since six months prior to the first test. Even then, you should be cautious about stopping safe sex; if you need to resume it in the future—for example, if you have a new partner—it may be a difficult readjustment to make.

Few in U.S. Need Testing for HIV-2

HIV-2 is a variant of HIV that is prevalent in western Africa. HIV-2 is transmitted through the same routes as HIV-1 and, like HIV-1, can cause AIDS. The HIV antibody test commonly available in the United States is a test for antibodies to HIV-1 and does not always detect infection with HIV-2. A small number of cases of HIV-2 infection have been reported in the United States. All identified HIV-2-infected U.S. residents have been immigrants from western Africa or their sexual partners.[9]

If any portion of your risk for HIV infection (from transfusion, needle sharing, or unprotected sexual contact) occurred in, or through a person coming from, a western African nation (including Guinea-Bissau, Ivory Coast, Senegal, Burkina Faso, Cape Verde Island), you should be tested not only for antibodies to HIV-1 but also for antibodies to HIV-2. See the Resource Guide for more information.

DISCRIMINATION RELATED TO TESTING

The HIV antibody test is not just a neutral medical test but has wide-ranging social and legal implications. It may be useful for you to know in advance whether you are positive or negative if you face mandatory HIV antibody testing related to employment.

The federal government requires all applicants for immigration to the United States and all employees and applicants to certain programs to take the HIV antibody test. These programs include the Peace Corps, the Foreign Service of the State Department, the armed forces, the state National Guard, and residential training programs of the Job Corps. Discrimination is practiced against those who test positive. Applicants for the Peace Corps and the Foreign Service who test positive are rejected. Current members of the foreign service who are positive or have spouses or dependent children who test positive are barred from most posts outside the United States. It is ironic that in following such practices, the government ignores the advice of its own public health officials.

If you allow the government to test you, your results will be part of official government records and not sufficiently confidential. Consequently, you should be anonymously tested before applying to join any such organization and should consider withdrawing your application if you are positive. See chapter 7, "Discrimination and Confidentiality."

Large-Scale Coercive Testing Programs Not Advisable

Many proposals for large-scale coercive HIV antibody testing programs have been suggested. Few of these proposals have been supported by responsible epidemiologists and public health officials.[10] The debate over coercive testing is often wrongly characterized as a conflict between the public health and the civil rights of HIV-infected people. This misconception rests on the false premise that coercive testing would prevent new infections. HIV can be transmitted by unsafe sexual activity and through needle sharing. Since these are voluntary behaviors, new infections through these routes could be entirely prevented by appropriate education and persuasion. Testing cannot stop new infections without the cooperation of the public. This cooperation can be attained through education and voluntary anonymous testing programs.

No Need for Testing in Work Settings

According to the U.S. Public Health Service, there is no reason anyone needs to be HIV antibody-tested to protect others at their place of employment, even if they work with children or in a health-care setting.

Home Testing

Sometime in 1995 or early 1996, the federal government will probably approve the availability of HIV testing that can be done at home. These tests will probably involve pricking yourself to obtain a small amount of blood. This blood will be sent to a laboratory for EIA and Western blot testing. Results will be given over the phone with some counseling. Home testing has been a matter of some controversy. The advantage of home testing is that it may increase the number of people who know that they are HIV-infected and thus seek appropriate medical care. The disadvantage is that counseling will be limited and positive results returned on the phone may produce psychological trauma.

5

Health Care

At some point, HIV infection will probably be a controllable disease—a serious, lifelong disease, but manageable, as diabetes usually is now. The major advances made in treatment of HIV disease are in prevention and treatment of opportunistic infections: *Pneumocystis carinii* pneumonia (PCP), the most common cause of death from AIDS, is now usually preventable. Several antiviral medications (AZT, ddI, ddC, 3TC, and D4T) are now available, and new classes of antiviral drugs are being researched. While much remains to be understood about how to use these drugs, it is clear that at least some of the current antivirals can delay progression of the disease and improve the health of people with AIDS. The life expectancy of people with AIDS has been increased through more accurate diagnosis; prevention of opportunistic infections; prompt, aggressive treatment of opportunistic infections; and, probably, through the use of antivirals.

If you are HIV-infected, it is important for your physician to monitor your immune system, since you may have serious immune deficiency and be at high risk of developing an AIDS-related infection or tumor in the near future even if you feel completely healthy. Treatments to prevent opportunistic infection often need to be started by people who are asymptomatic or only mildly symptomatic.

The decision about when to start treating HIV disease with antiviral drugs is currently a matter of scientific debate and personal decision. In the future, with the development of new and better drugs, the hope is that HIV infection may be treated before serious damage to the immune system and the development of symptoms.

HIV TREATMENT IN CONTEXT

As research on AIDS and HIV infection progresses, options for therapy change rapidly. Physicians not directly involved in caring for people with AIDS are not generally able to keep up with all the information necessary to provide the best possible care to HIV-infected people.

Effective treatment relies on accurate diagnosis, which is difficult because a single symptom or illness may be caused by a variety of infectious organisms. For example, diarrhea may be caused by organisms such as cryptosporidia, cytomegalovirus (CMV), *Mycobacterium avium* (MAC), microsporidia, and many others.[1] Some of these can easily be treated with medication and some are difficult to treat. Also, specific organisms may respond to specific medications.[2, 3, 4] Conversely, a single infectious organism may cause a variety of symptoms and illnesses. For example, CMV can cause diarrhea, encephalitis, or infection of the retina.[5]

A health care provider knowledgeable about AIDS is in the best position to diagnose HIV-related illness. An expert is also in the best position to tell you when a physical change is not an HIV-related symptom and will consequently be better able to give you credible and comforting reassurance.

Join the HIV Information Network

If you are HIV-infected, get information from people who are in a similar situation. Support groups for HIV-infected people and lectures on treatment are conducted by AIDS service organizations, clinics, hospitals, and particularly by organizations established by and run for people with AIDS. The AIDS treatment movement is an informal collection of individuals and organizations who research and publicize treatments for HIV-related illness. In some cases, buyers' groups supply substances for the treatment of HIV-related illness. Good sources of information tend to be concentrated in cities with large populations of HIV-infected people. You can also learn about treatment by subscribing to the treatment newsletters listed in the Resource Guide.

Practice Risk Reduction

Treatment should be combined with risk reduction. Use of condoms for intercourse prevents the transmission of other diseases that may cause serious illness in people with HIV. This includes transmission of certain opportunistic infections that are not always seen as being sexually transmitted but probably are. These include KS, cryptosporidium, and microsporidium. Repeated exposure to HIV or infection with other sexually transmitted diseases may also help to trigger illness in people who are infected but otherwise healthy. Guidelines given in chapter 3 can help you minimize your risk from sexual activity or needle-sharing.

Psychosocial Obstacles to Good Care

A subtle set of obstacles to getting good care stems from the inevitable, understandable interference of your emotions in the complex decisions you will be called upon to make. Fear of AIDS and a reluctance to think about the topic may make it difficult for you to absorb the information you need to make decisions rationally. You may put all thoughts of AIDS out of your mind, perhaps feeling that if you don't think about AIDS, you won't get sick. "Positive thinking" is a dangerous attitude if it interferes with your getting adequate medical care. It is easy to imagine that seeing your doctor regularly or taking medication—becoming a "patient"—might make you feel that you are sick. In practice, many people feel relieved after seeing an expert physician or after beginning treatment.

The pessimism and fatalism surrounding AIDS as reported in the media may encourage you to adopt a passive attitude. A variety of complex social and psychological factors may cause people who are HIV-infected to feel guilty. This is not surprising in a society where people with AIDS are frequently blamed for their illness. If guilt or pessimism stops you from getting the best possible medical care, get help from an HIV support group, concerned friends, or a psychotherapist.

HEALTH CARE STRATEGIES FOR HIV-INFECTED PEOPLE

Finding an Expert Doctor

Get medical care from a doctor who is knowledgeable about HIV-related issues. If you have good health-insurance coverage, it may be relatively easy to find a suitable private doctor. However, if limited insurance means that you have to rely on clinic, health maintenance organization (HMO), or medicaid services, your choices will be more restricted. Drugs, therapies, tests, and procedures can also be too expensive for the individual to finance out-of-pocket.

Get Referrals

To find a physician, call a local AIDS organization and ask for referrals. Ask friends and acquaintances for their experiences, good and bad, with recommended doctors. If there are no AIDS organizations near you, try calling a local gay political or social group, which might have such information. You can also call a major medical center in or near your community, particularly one associated with a medical school, and ask for the names of health care providers who are knowledgeable about HIV infection and AIDS. Ask to speak to someone in the infectious disease or internal medicine departments. Multiple sources of information that confirm each other are the most reliable. For example, if a physician is recommended by an AIDS organization and a hospital and is liked by several friends, it is probable you have located a good source of treatment. Your research will ultimately pay off in better medical care.

There is currently a shortage of doctors expert in AIDS. Some expert doctors have full practices and cannot take new patients. However, they should be able to refer you to other expert doctors.

Local Doctors May Not Be Expert in AIDS

Most large cities will have some physicians expert in the diagnosis and treatment of HIV disease. If you live in a small town or rural area and you can afford it, go to a nearby major city for a consultation with an expert physician. The doctor you consult and your own local health care provider should communicate by telephone or mail after the consultation.

If You Cannot Choose a Private Physician

If you belong to a health maintenance organization (HMO, see chapter 6, "Insurance"), your choice of physicians will be limited to those working for the HMO. Call the HMO and ask for the names of any doctors on their panel who are

AIDS experts. Call an AIDS organization and friends to ask for further information about these doctors. If you rely on medicaid, go to a clinic specifically set up to care for people with HIV-related illnesses. Some major cities (New York, San Francisco, Los Angeles) have such clinics, often associated with major hospitals. You may have to rely on medical care from a hospital without a special HIV-clinic program. It is still best to choose a hospital with some reputation for treating AIDS patients: doctors in such facilities are likely to know the most about the medical care you need.

Doctors Will Not Solve All Your Problems

It is reasonable to try out more than one doctor, if time and money allow and this is not too stressful. A good match between doctor and patient probably depends on a number of subtle factors. However, if you see several doctors and have strong objections to all of them, you may need to change your expectations. Many people feel anxious or frightened about seeing doctors, and the nervousness may be heightened when the visit concerns an HIV-related matter.

There are many questions about HIV illness that no doctor can answer. At times you may even bring your doctor new articles or information to be evaluated. You may have an understandable desire for definite answers where none exist. A variety of emotional needs accrue around the topic of illness: unconsciously, you may want something from your doctor that no doctor can provide.

Make the Best Use of Visits to Your Doctor

Prepare before visiting your doctor. Write down a list of questions you want to ask. Without a list, you may get nervous and forget what you intended to ask. If possible, discuss your questions with a sympathetic and knowledgeable friend. Anxiety during visits to your doctor may be reduced by having a friend accompany you.

Your visits to your doctor may take place under rushed circumstances, but you are entitled to take time to ask questions and discuss issues. Some expert physicians are so busy caring for people severely ill with AIDS that they have little time left over to care for those who are less ill. Ideally, physicians should have enough time to talk to patients about the problems of HIV-related illness. In actuality, you have to be realistic about the pressures of doctors' schedules—you should always expect to do some waiting. However, if you find that your doctor never has time to answer questions, get another doctor, if possible.

Make sure your physician understands your concern for confidentiality (see chapter 7, "Discrimination and Confidentiality"). Discuss what information will be recorded in your medical records, and how that information may best be protected.

Initial Doctor's Visit

When you first go to be evaluated, your doctor will want to get a good general picture of your health by taking a medical history, performing a physical examination, and ordering laboratory tests. This initial workup will form a baseline useful for future reference.

History and Physical

Be prepared to list illnesses you have had in the past with approximate dates and any medications you were given. Mention infectious diseases you have had (such as sexually transmitted diseases or hepatitis B) and also any allergies—especially to medications. Tell your doctor about other medications and drugs you may be taking, including nonmedical drugs such as alcohol and other recreational drugs. The physical examination may include a close inspection for skin problems common in HIV infection. Your doctor will probably also check for enlarged lymph nodes, mouth ulcers and sores, and genital problems.

General Laboratory Tests

Standard blood tests are used to determine your general health status and uncover any active disease processes in your body. Common tests include a complete blood count (CBC), platelet count, and a "differential," which counts the different types of white blood cells. You may be tested for specific diseases: hepatitis B, syphilis, tuberculosis, chlamydia, gonorrhea (genital, rectal, and pharyngeal sites), and intestinal parasites.

Immune System Evaluation

Physicians frequently order lymphocyte subsets or subpopulation studies (often called T-cell tests) to test the immune system of new HIV-infected patients. Lymphocyte subset studies are blood tests done on a small sample drawn from the arm. Lymphocytes are one type of white blood cell.

Two kinds of lymphocytes are of most concern: CD4 cells (or helper cells, also referred to as T4 cells) and CD8 cells (or suppressor cells, also referred to as T8 cells). CD4 cells are the part of the immune system that helps other immune cells (B cells) produce antibodies to fight viral, fungal, and parasitic infections. CD8 cells eradicate cancerous, infected, defective, immature, or superfluous cells from the body. Sometimes CD8 cells eliminate cells that were mass-produced to fight off infections, but which the body no longer needs.

HIV infects and destroys CD4 cells, gradually reducing the total number of these cells in the bodies of HIV-infected people. There appear to be multiple mechanisms by which HIV kills CD4 cells. HIV also infects other cells in the immune system and appears to cause a variety of abnormalities.

The results of lymphocyte subset studies can be expressed in several ways. The absolute CD4 count measures the number of CD4 cells in a standard volume of blood (usually expressed in cells per cubic millimeter). The CD4 percent measures the percent of all lymphocytes that are

CD4 cells. The CD4:CD8 ratio measures the relative numbers of these cells. Most clinical studies have used the absolute CD4 count as a marker to measure the functioning of the immune system.

Non-HIV-infected healthy people usually have results in the following range:

- CD4 cells range from 500 to 1,600 cells per cubic millimeter
- CD4 percents range from 40% to 70%
- CD4:CD8 ratios range from 1.0 to 4.0

Many people with HIV have CD4 counts that are lower than this, but most illnesses do not develop unless CD4 counts are below 200. A single test result should not be taken to be conclusive. The CD4 count is a volatile measure, analogous to your pulse rate. Just as exercise can raise your pulse and resting can slow it down, the degree of challenge to your immune system can change your CD4 count rapidly in either direction. CD4 counts in an individual vary over a day. Counts performed on two blood samples drawn from the same person twelve hours apart may differ widely, occasionally by as much as 50% (several hundred cells). Laboratory technique can also affect CD4 cell counts; if your blood is tested at different laboratories, your results may vary. Other things that temporarily affect your CD4 count include other illnesses, sleep deprivation, alcohol, and other drug use. The overall trend over months of time is more significant than any single number.

Prognostic Tests in Development

CD4 cell tests are useful as an indicator of when the development of opportunistic infections may occur. However, people who take antiviral drugs may get small rises in CD4 counts. These rises are not permanent and may not be a reliable measure of clinical benefit of the drug.

Tests not yet widely used may in the future add to the

predictive power of the CD4 cell count. New tests that count the amount of HIV RNA (strips of genetic material) may add to the predictive power of CD4 counts or even replace them as a direct marker of the progression of disease.[6] These tests are sometimes referred to as viral-load tests.

At least two such tests, Chiron's branch-chained DNA (bDNA) and Hoffmann–La Roche's HIV RNA quantitative PCR, use different techniques but produce similar results on the same sample of blood. Other companies are developing similar tests. These tests measure the number of viral particles per milliliter of blood.

There is uncertainty about how to use these tests to understand the course of illness and plan treatment. Further studies are being conducted. So far, studies suggest that in most people, as levels of the virus increase, their health deteriorates, and that people stay healthy when the viral load is low.[7] Some strains of the virus may be more harmful to the body than others, which may add a further complication to interpreting these results.

It is likely that, in the near future, measuring viral load will show when to start antiviral therapy or switch from one antiviral drug to another. Although there are no clear-cut guidelines yet, expert clinicians often look at a combination of CD4 cell count and viral load to make recommendations about antiviral drugs.

Routine Care and Immune-Function Monitoring

You and your physician should decide on a regular schedule of routine visits. If you are HIV-infected and have no symptoms, you should see your physician at least every six months. If you have significant symptoms or AIDS, you should schedule more frequent appointments.

Immune-Function Monitoring

HIV-infected patients should have immune-function tests done at least two to four times per year. Unfortunately, lymphocyte subset studies are quite expensive and may cost several hundred dollars each time they are performed; health care insurance including medicaid pays for these tests. If paying for your laboratory tests is a problem, ask your physician to request only a CD4-cell count or CD4- and CD8-cell count rather than the complete set of lymphocyte subset studies—the cost will be considerably less.

Tests of viral load are still considered experimental. They cost about $200; health insurance and medicaid may not always pay for these tests.

If the results of immune-function tests suggest significant immune impairment (CD4 cell count below 200), you should begin preventive drug therapy (prophylaxis) against opportunistic infections such as PCP. On the basis of current studies, expert physicians disagree about whether patients should start antivirals when their CD4 cells are between 200 and 500.

Immunization

HIV-infected people should protect themselves from infections that may weaken the immune system. Vaccination can protect against infections, but vaccination itself may constitute a small challenge to the immune system. Challenging the immune system may not always be a good idea because it stimulates proliferation of CD4 cells, which, if these cells are infected with HIV, also stimulates the multiplication of the virus.

Vaccines are not all alike. Live-virus or live-bacterial vaccines contain weakened but still active forms of the microorganism against which you are being inoculated. Live vaccines such as oral attenuated polio vaccine (OPV) should generally not be given to HIV-infected people who have symptoms of immune suppression. Some travel vaccines such as that for yellow fever are live vaccines. In some cases it is possible to substitute immune globulins (which confer temporary protection against an illness) for a live-virus vaccine.

Some vaccines have been completely inactivated as disease-causing agents and are referred to as killed vaccines. Killed-virus vaccines are thought to be safe. They include hepatitis A vaccine, hepatitis B vaccine, influenza vaccine, inactivated polio vaccine (IPV), pneumococcal vaccine, diptheria-tetanus vaccine, injected typhoid vaccine, and Haemophilus B vaccine. It is recommended that all people at risk for HIV receive pneumococcal vaccine (pneumovax), a series of three hepatitis B vaccinations, as well as an influenza vaccination each year (around October). Some physicians also recommend haemophilus B vaccine and hepatitis A vaccine for people with HIV.

HIV-infected children should receive inactivated polio vaccine (IPV) rather than oral attenuated polio vaccine (OPV) as well as the regular schedule of other immunizations.[8] Uninfected children living in a household with an immune-deficient adult should receive IPV rather than OPV so that the children do not shed polio-virus particles that might harm the adult.

Hepatitis B Vaccine

Hepatitis B is a dangerous disease in its own right and may complicate the development of HIV disease. If you contract hepatitis B, you can become a chronic carrier and risk developing serious liver disease. Those at greatest risk for hepatitis B are needle-sharers, health care workers, men who have had sex with men, and the sexual partners of these people. A vaccine for hepatitis B is available to protect those at risk. This vaccine has no serious side effects and is now given to newborn children. Contrary to rumor, there is no danger of contracting HIV infection through hepatitis B vaccination.[9]

Hepatitis A Vaccine

In early 1995, a new hepatitis A vaccine was licensed for use in the United States. Hepatitis A, although less serious than Hepatitis B, can cause significant illness. It is common in sexually active adults, even when they practice safer sex. You should discuss the need for this vaccine with your physician.

Check for Tuberculosis

People who are infected with HIV are more susceptible to tuberculosis (TB), probably because HIV infection may allow a latent (that is, inactive) TB infection to become reactivated. If you are positive on a TB test and do not know your HIV antibody status, you should also be HIV antibody tested. Also, if you are HIV-infected, you should be tested for TB. Special diagnostic studies may be needed to diagnose TB in patients who are HIV-infected.[10] HIV-infected people may require a nonstandard course of treatment for TB as well as careful monitoring for adverse reactions and evaluation for signs of relapse after therapy is completed.[11]

Gynecological and Obstetrical Issues

Inadequate data is available regarding women with AIDS. Most studies have focused on men with AIDS. HIV disease in women is complicated by the fact that most infected women in the United States are poor women of color. Their access to medical care is poor, and other social factors work against adequate treatment. Women often neglect their health care needs because of the burden of caring for children. Diagnosis is often made relatively late due to both limited medical care and the failure of physicians to identify symptoms of HIV disease in women.

The higher death rate in women with AIDS is probably a reflection of these factors.[12] It is not yet known whether biological factors also play a role. In studies so far, the natural history of the disease seems similar to that in men: AIDS-defining illnesses occur at the same level of CD4 count.[13]

In 1992, the definition of AIDS was expanded. Several diseases specific to women were included in this expanded definition: cancer of the cervix, vulvovaginal candidiasis, cervical dysplasia, and pelvic inflammatory disease. All of these diseases occur in noninfected women but appear to occur at a higher rate in HIV-infected women.[14]

Women who are HIV-infected may be more prone to cervical disorders than uninfected women. Some expert clinicians have recommended that an initial exam include colposcopy (magnified visual inspection of the cervix) in addition to a Pap smear, followed by a Pap smear every six months.[15]

Although it was initially thought that pregnancy might increase an HIV-infected woman's risk of developing symptoms, recent studies contradict this.[16] The pregnancy of an infected woman has a 15 to 40% chance of resulting in a baby born with HIV infection.[17] Appropriate use of AZT and other interventions lower the risk further.

If you are a pregnant woman who is HIV-infected, you may want to seek counseling about whether to continue the pregnancy. If you carry the fetus to term, get obstetrical care from a physician who is extremely knowledgeable about HIV infection. Pregnancy may necessitate the modification of standard treatment regimes because some drugs used in treating HIV-related illnesses may cross the placental barrier and adversely affect the fetus.[18]

Since newborns may be infected through drinking breast milk, do not plan to breast-feed (many substitutes for breast milk are available). Since newborns carry their mother's antibodies, all infants born to HIV-infected mothers will initially test positive for HIV antibodies, but only some are actually infected.[19]

Medication

Discuss the use of all prescription and over-the-counter medications with your physician. Even commonly used nonprescription drugs may occasionally cause problems for those who are HIV-infected. For example, aspirin can be dangerous for people with low platelet count, a condition that more commonly occurs in people with HIV infection.[20, 21]

Bodybuilders who want to increase muscle mass sometimes take steroids without a doctor's prescription. This practice can be dangerous, as steroids can cause liver and other organ damage. Also, sharing equipment for injecting steroids can transmit HIV just as easily as sharing equipment for injecting heroin. However, low doses of anabolic steroids may be a useful treatment for severe weight loss and diminished sexual interest and function in people with AIDS.[22] Doctors can legally prescribe therapeutic doses of these drugs.

You should also inform your doctor about your alcohol, marijuana, or other recreational-drug use. Recreational drugs may conflict with the drugs that your doctor prescribes. For example, one alcoholic drink, or even cough syrup with alcohol, can cause severe nausea when combined with some medications.

If you smoke marijuana, sterilize it in the oven (low temperature for five minutes) or the microwave (high setting for one minute). This kills spores in the marijuana that cause a life-threatening infection called aspergillosis. Marijuana seems to have medicinal properties, as a treatment for nausea and lack of appetite.

Symptoms of HIV-Related Illness

Remember that HIV disease takes many different courses. Symptoms that appear in HIV disease are common to many illnesses and not specific for HIV disease. The first noticeable symptoms of HIV-related illness are often the same as the symptoms of many common ailments such as colds and flu. Some of these symptoms can also be caused by anxiety or depression.

Other Advice

If you have AIDS or HIV infection, you can protect your health in many small ways. Regular exercise, adequate sleep, and stress reduction are important components in maintaining health.

Eat a sensible, well-balanced diet. Consult with a nutritionist knowledgeable about HIV infection, especially if you are losing weight or having gastrointestinal symptoms. Cook all meats to the medium stage or more. Do not eat raw beef, raw fish, or uncooked eggs—these foods may be contaminated with bacteria or parasites. If you travel to areas where sanitary conditions are poor, be especially cautious about what you eat and drink.[23] If in doubt, always drink bottled water or carbonated beverages.

In the United States, water supplies in a number of areas have recently been shown to be infected with cryptosporidium and other organisms that may cause harm to people with HIV disease. There are three possible ways to avoid this danger:

- You can boil all drinking water.
- You can buy bottled water. Not all bottled water is free of harmful organisms; only some brands are regularly monitored for cryptosporidium. Bottled water from commercial reverse-osmosis plants is safe. Bottled distilled water is always safe.
- You can also purchase a water filter to use at home. Not all filters will eliminate cryptosporidium. The most effective are those employing reverse osmosis and those certified by a group called NSF International under its standard 53. Filters must be labeled "absolute one micron." You can obtain more specific information by call-

ing the CDC national AIDS information line (800-342-2437).

People with AIDS seem to be depleted of certain essential vitamins and minerals. This deficiency may start early in the infection. You may get blood tests from your physician that will indicate whether you are deficient in specific vitamins. Vitamins and minerals that seem to be particularly important to HIV-infected people are vitamin B_{12}, folate, selenium, and antioxidants.

Taking a daily vitamin supplement may be useful and will not harm you. If you take high doses of any vitamins, discuss this with your doctor, as some vitamins may be harmful in high doses.

Avoid infections that may be passed through the wastes of birds, rodents, reptiles, and insects. Such wastes are often found in old, dusty, or dirty areas. Since cat feces can be contaminated with the dangerous parasite *Toxoplasma gondii*, HIV-infected people should wear rubber gloves when cleaning out a cat's litter box.[24]

TREATMENT AND PREVENTION OF OPPORTUNISTIC INFECTIONS

Good patient management for HIV-infected people requires close monitoring of the patient's health so that prompt diagnosis and active intervention can be made in all the varied medical problems that come up in HIV-related illness. Good patient management is critical in maintaining the health of those who are HIV-infected and extending the life span and improving the quality of life of people with AIDS.

Infections Should Be Treated Promptly and Aggressively

Some people who are HIV-infected and developing immune impairment will develop one or more relatively minor infections. Evidence indicates that it is important to treat these infections quickly and thoroughly because ongoing infection may put a strain on the immune system and worsen the course of HIV infection. HIV-infected people may need to be treated with longer courses of medication or higher dosages than patients not infected with HIV.[25] Also, those who are HIV-infected more often have adverse reactions to medication.

Inform your doctor if you develop any symptoms or reactions to medication. It is understandable that you may be anxious about even minor symptoms if you know you are HIV-infected, and you should be able to discuss them with your physician. Your psychological peace of mind is important, as is early intervention in any medical problems.

Pneumocystis Carinii Pneumonia (PCP) Can Be Prevented

It is always better to prevent an illness rather than to treat it after it has occurred. Certain medications are now being effectively used to prevent episodes of PCP, particularly a mixture of two antibiotics called sulfamethoxazole and trimethoprim (trade-named Bactrim or Septra). Other drugs that are used but which are less effective for prevention of PCP are dapsone,[26] pentamidine,[27] and Mepron.[28]

The U.S. Public Health Service has officially recommended that physicians offer primary preventive treatment for PCP to all HIV-infected people with a CD4 cell count below 200 (or if CD4 lymphocytes form less than 20% of total lymphocytes).[29] This also applies to those people already taking antivirals, as antivirals alone do not provide sufficient protection against PCP. Some physicians begin PCP prevention when the CD4 count drops below 250 rather than 200.

HIV-infected people frequently become allergic to sulfa-based drugs such as Bactrim. The symptoms of this allergy are fever, hives, itchiness, and an extensive rash. These symptoms disappear when Bactrim is discontinued. The allergy can often be controlled through desensitization (re-challenge or dose escalation in tiny amounts), sometimes in combination with antihistamine and anti-inflammatory medication.[30] Those unable to tolerate Bactrim can use one of the other drugs that prevent PCP.

A number of other drugs have become available for prophylaxis of other opportunistic diseases. For example, Bactrim may prevent toxoplasmosis and some bacterial infection as well as PCP.[31] Acyclovir can prevent herpes outbreaks; higher doses of this drug may prevent shingles. Fluconazole or itraconazole may prevent the development of severe fungal infections.[32] Rifabutin, clarithromycin, and azithromycin can prevent MAC. Oral ganciclovir and valaciclovir prevent the development of CMV.[33]

However, taking a drug to prevent the development of an opportunistic infection may not always be the best thing to do. Toxicity may outweigh the benefits of some drugs. Resistance to drugs may develop, making future treatment for active infection more difficult. For example, rifabutin and clarithromycin are now available to prevent MAC. However, if these drugs are started at preventive doses when someone has an undiagnosed MAC infection, resistance may occur, and options for treatment of the infection will be limited.[34]

One drug alone is not sufficient to prevent some diseases. Careful clinical evaluation, including assessment of an individual's risk for a particular infection, is necessary before starting any medication.

FDA-APPROVED AND EXPERIMENTAL DRUGS

Types of Drug Treatments

In addition to drugs used to treat opportunistic infections and malignancies, two main classes of drugs are available for primary therapy of HIV-infection: antiviral drugs and immunomodulators. Some drugs belong to both these classes.

Antiviral Drugs

Antiviral drugs are directed against HIV itself, rather than against some consequence of the infection. Some antiviral drugs prevent infection of cells with HIV, and some prevent infected cells from producing new virus. Some that are currently being researched may reduce the capacity of the virus to cause harm to the immune system.

There are many unanswered questions about antiviral therapy, including when to begin drugs, which drugs to use, and whether to use a combination of drugs. However, there is general agreement that it is important to start using antiviral medication in the following circumstances: if your CD4 cell count falls below 200, if there is a rapid sustained decrease in CD4 cells or a rapid sustained increase in viral load, or if you have developed an opportunistic infection. All of the antiviral drugs currently available have been shown to produce short-term improvements in CD4 cells and viral load.

The United States Food and Drug Administration (FDA) has approved five antiviral drugs. These drugs are:

- AZT (azidothymidine)
- ddI (dideoxyinosine)
- ddC (dideoxycytidine)

- D4T (stavudine)
- 3TC (lamivudine).

All of these drugs belong to the category of antivirals named nucleoside analogues, which operate by disrupting the synthesis of viral DNA.

AZT and ddI were the first antiviral drugs approved, and consequently more information about how to use these particular antivirals is available.[35] AZT and ddI have been shown to decrease the occurrence of opportunistic infections in people with AIDS and to slow the progression of disease in people with fewer than 500 CD4 cells.[36, 37, 38, 39]

Many controversies surround the use of AZT, ddI, and the other antiviral drugs. All of these drugs seem to work only for a short time, then HIV develops resistance. There may be cumulative side effects to these drugs. Drugs are currently being approved on the basis of changes in CD4 count and viral load, so-called surrogate markers. There is disagreement about how well these markers correlate with the development of illnesses associated with HIV and with survival time for an individual. This is an important area for discussion with your physician when you are considering antiviral treatment.

When to Start

When to start antiviral drugs is a complicated issue that can be addressed only briefly here. There is no certainty about the best course of action, information from clinical trials is incomplete and contradictory, and the situation changes as new drugs are developed. For this reason, it is important to consult with a physician who is up-to-date and to try to stay well-informed about new developments.

Following are current generally accepted recommendations about when to start antivirals:[40]

- For people with CD4 cells above 500, the use of antivirals is empiric (done without proof of effectiveness). They are generally not recommended, but experts have varying opinions.

- For people whose CD4 cells are between 200 and 500 and have no serious symptoms, the current guideline from the National Institute of Allergies and Infectious Diseases (NIAID) is that you have a choice of initiating antiviral treatment or waiting until CD4 cells are lower or certain symptoms develop.[41, 42] Many physicians note that patients with CD4 cell counts above 200 have a better response to drugs and that it is better to keep the immune system functioning well, especially since several antivirals are available and new drugs are being developed. However, other experts suggest that only AZT and ddI have been shown to have a clinical benefit in people with AIDS. Since the available antivirals may only work for a limited time (one to two years), some experts think that the benefit of antivirals should be saved for later in the illness.

- The NIAID does recommend that all patients with CD4 counts below 200 and those with higher counts and serious symptoms use some antiviral(s). However, no clinical studies have proven the effectiveness of antiviral drugs for people with very low CD4 cells (below 50).

Using Available Antivirals

Antiviral drugs can be used alone or in combination. Conclusive information is lacking about which drug(s) to start first and which combinations of drugs are useful. For example, AZT and ddC may work better than either drug alone in people with 50 to 300 CD4 cells, but may be worse than AZT alone in people with less than 50 CD4 cells.

Combinations that many experts recommend include:

- AZT and ddI
- AZT and ddC
- AZT and 3TC

There is at least some data that each of these combinations produces a transient increase in CD4 cells and a decrease in viral load. There is no proof of long-term clinical efficacy. Some experts also recommend the use of DT4 with either ddI or 3TC.

All of the currently available antiviral drugs can have some severe side effects, such as bone-marrow suppression (leading to anemia and low white blood cell counts)[43] and peripheral neuropathy. These side effects are often reversible by stopping the drug, reducing the dose, or using other drugs to treat the side effects.

Approved antivirals are generally expensive drugs. Insurance policies that cover medication pay for AZT, as does medicaid. Some special state programs help those who are not medicaid-eligible afford antivirals: see the Resource Guide.

Newer Antivirals

Protease Inhibitors

Protease inhibitors belong to a different class of antivirals from nucleoside analogues. They are designed to keep infected cells from producing new virus.[44] A number of pharmaceutical companies have such drugs in development, and it seems highly likely that they will have a role in treating HIV disease. Some people are taking these drugs as part of a clinical trial, and they are available from drug companies to people who cannot tolerate or no longer benefit from approved antiviral drugs.

Protease inhibitors dramatically reduce levels of HIV, temporarily, and boost CD4 cell counts. However, in the protease inhibitors now in clinical trials, resistance eventually occurs and the drug stops working, at least in people with higher levels of virus.[45] Some of these drugs reduce viral load more than AZT and other nucleoside analogues and may be less toxic.[46] None of them seems to be a "magic bullet," that is, a single drug that when used alone cures the disease.

We do not know whether combining protease inhibitors with other available drugs increases their effectiveness, but it is an encouraging possibility. We do not know whether these drugs should be used late in disease or early. Well-designed studies may give us the answers.

A number of other antiviral drugs that hinder the virus in varied ways are in development. Some of the categories of drugs you may hear about are:

- TAT gene inhibitors and LTR blockers, which force the virus to remain latent in infected cells
- gene therapies, a category that actually describes a number of different antiviral therapies
- integrase drugs
- antisense drugs
- non-nucleoside reverse transcriptase inhibitors (nnrti) such as nevirapine and delaviridine

Immune Modulators

Immune modulators are drugs that help control the effects of HIV either by stimulating positive changes in the immune system or by suppressing negative changes.

An example of an immune modulator is IL-2, also known as interleukin-2. IL-2 is a manufactured version of a chemical found in the body that stimulates the production of CD4 cells. Currently, there is not enough evidence to tell whether these drugs will be clinically useful. In addition, in people with less than 200 CD4 cells, IL-2 seems to stimulate the growth of the virus more than it produces new CD4 cells. IL-2 also has significant side effects.[47] IL-2 is available by prescription, but it is expensive and its use in people with HIV (outside of trials) is highly speculative.

Other immune-modulator drugs that are currently being studied include other interleukins, interferons, immunoglobulins, monoclonal antibodies, thymic hormones, antioxidants, and anti-inflammatories.

All of these drugs are in relatively early development. Some may be helpful, others may cause more harm than good. If you are going to take an experimental drug, you must obtain up-to-date information about what is known about the benefits and costs of the drug.

ACCESS TO EXPERIMENTAL TREATMENTS

Clinical trials are under way to test the efficacy of dozens of experimental drugs in preventing illness in people with asymptomatic HIV infection as well as people with symptoms or AIDS. Inform yourself about the current status of clinical trials and the availability of experimental drugs. HIV-infected people have gained access to experimental therapies through participation as subjects in clinical trials, importation of drugs from other countries, or purchase through AIDS-treatment buyers' groups.

Clinical Drug Trials

The safety and efficacy of new drugs can only be scientifically proven through controlled clinical studies. In a controlled study, subjects are divided into two groups: one group receives the drug being tested; another group, called the control group, does not receive the drug.

Sometimes the control group is given an inactive substitute called a placebo, and sometimes another drug whose properties are known. It is necessary to control studies in order to know whether the drug under trial is responsible for any beneficial changes observed in the subjects. However, if a particular drug for an illness has been proved safe and effective, trials of other drugs for the same illness may be compared to the proven drug.

In a double-blind controlled study neither the subjects nor the researchers know which subject is receiving the real drug and which is getting the substitute. Double-blind studies are useful because it has been shown that researchers and subjects may unconsciously bias a study toward the desired conclusion if they know what treatment they are receiving.

Sources of information about clinical drug trials for AIDS and HIV infection are listed in the Resource Guide. To decide whether to become a subject in a clinical trial, consider the following questions:

- Do you trust the researchers? Are they affiliated with a reputable research institution or do they have a respected board of directors? Do they have a good reputation among people with AIDS and with the gay community?
- If the study is double-blind, will the researchers break the double-blind code if the control group appears to be doing significantly better or worse than the group receiving treatment? This should be part of the informed-consent form you will be asked to sign.
- Do the expected medical benefits to you outweigh the risk of adverse side effects?
- Do the expected benefits outweigh the chance that you may receive the drug at an inadequate dose and develop resistance to a potentially useful drug?
- Will the researchers allow you to take treatments or drugs other than those under study in the trial?
- Will your confidentiality be protected?
- Will the drug be provided after termination of the trial? If so, at what cost (if any)?
- Will the study provide counseling or other psychological support for subjects?
- Will you get any benefits from participation other than receiving the drug under study? (Examples of such benefits are specialized medical care or free laboratory testing.)
- Will you be able to get access to all medical data collected

on you? Will you get access to diagnostic or prognostic tests not available to the general public?

Drug trials recruit subjects who meet entry criteria— that is, who fit various medical and demographic profiles. For example, some trials will accept only subjects with AIDS while others accept only those with milder symptoms. Some trials exclude women and children, and many trials explicitly exclude IV drug users.

Drugs Available through the Expanded Access Program and Compassionate Use and Treatment IND Protocols

Those who cannot get access to experimental drugs through clinical trials because they do not fit the inclusion criteria or because they live too far away from the site of trials may be able to obtain some drugs through what is known as expanded access. The advantage of expanded access is that it gives individuals a wider choice of drugs to use.

People who fit specific criteria—often people who are very ill—may sometimes be able to get unproven drugs from pharmaceutical companies under what are known as compassionate use and treatment IND protocols. These include both antivirals and drugs used to prevent and treat opportunistic infections and cancers. The drugs are usually provided without charge. Talk to your physician for more information.

Substances Available in Other Countries or through Buyers' Clubs

Because of differences in the regulation and approval processes in other countries, some drugs may first become available outside the United States. This has been true particularly for drugs used to treat or prevent opportunistic infections. For example, fluconazole, itraconazole, and albendazole were available in Europe to treat opportunistic infections long before their approval in the United States. Nonprofit buyers' clubs and AIDS treatment activist groups have been able to help people obtain some drugs from other countries. These groups have also imported certain FDA-approved medications at lower cost than that of the same medications in the United States. The PWA Health Group in New York City or Project Inform in San Francisco (both listed in the Resource Guide) can provide more information.

Criteria for Considering Experimental Treatment

Taking any substance that has not been shown to be safe through large-scale, controlled clinical trials means taking a risk. Any drug may have adverse side effects, particularly in people with impaired immune systems.[48] Given the gravity of the prognosis for seriously symptomatic HIV infection, some people have decided to risk taking untested (and possibly useless) medications. The problem is complex; there are no definitive answers about the effectiveness or dangers of using these drugs. The following principles may help you to decide whether to take a drug not yet proven safe or effective in the HIV setting:

- Is there some theoretical basis for hoping the drug may be effective against AIDS or HIV infection? Are test-tube studies encouraging?
- Is there a body of anecdotal evidence from clinicians or HIV-infected people in the AIDS treatment movement supporting the use of the drug?
- Is the drug known to have adverse side effects or to be toxic? Taking an unproven drug may cause harm instead of benefit. Evidence suggesting a drug is safe for use against HIV may be based on experience with the drug in

other settings. Some experimental therapies tried against HIV infection are FDA-approved for other uses.
- Is the drug known to interfere with any effective therapy you are currently taking? Your physician can help you answer this question.

Your physician cannot recommend unproven treatments but may be willing to advise you about the efficacy and safety of treatments you yourself suggest.

It is unfortunate but true that treatment for HIV infection will probably advance in small increments, rather than through discovery of one wonder drug. If someone tries to sell you a total cure for AIDS, watch out: people who face serious illness make easy targets for fraud. If the only support for a proposed treatment comes from the people who stand to profit from its use, be skeptical. Fraud of this type has been reported frequently.

PSYCHOLOGICAL FACTORS

AIDS has a particularly complex psychological dimension because it taps three great reservoirs of conflict: sex, death, and difference. The epidemic has done severe psychological as well as physical harm, causing anxiety and depression among people infected and at risk. It has also caused great upheaval in the social and sexual lives of millions of Americans.

The first step to combat psychological problems around HIV infection is to recognize your anxiety or depression. Worry about AIDS can manifest itself in various ways.:

- Preoccupation with AIDS to a degree that interferes with daily life. Those who actually have AIDS are not likely to be able to avoid such preoccupation.
- Denying worry about the illness while acting in a way that may lead to infection.

- Guilt, shame, or lowered self-esteem, particularly around the issues of sexuality or sexual orientation.
- Fear of infection of self or others in situations where no danger exists, such as casual contact.

Minor physical symptoms such as occasional diarrhea, a transient bruise, or a slight cough may trigger extreme anxiety. Minimize this anxiety by seeking the most sensitive medical care available to you. If you are made to feel that you are bothering your doctor when you ask detailed questions or present minor symptoms, try to find a health care provider who understands that appropriate reassurance and education are part of good medical care.

Talking with others who are also worried about HIV infection has helped many people. Actively working with AIDS political and service organizations to fight the epidemic can reduce feelings of powerlessness and isolation.

Sometimes people develop more severe psychological symptoms around the topic of AIDS. These include:

- persistent sadness or hopelessness
- intense nervousness or irritability
- anxiety attacks or panic attacks
- obsessive preoccupation with illness or physical symptoms
- increased use of drugs, including alcohol
- prolonged insomnia
- inability to concentrate, feelings of being "slowed down," loss of energy
- inability to function at work or at home
- inability to enjoy social or sexual life
- avoiding necessary medical care
- thoughts of suicide

If you are suffering any persistent combination of these symptoms, seek psychological counseling. Antidepressant medication can treat both anxiety and depression in people with HIV. If you are upset or worried that you might harm yourself, go to the emergency room of your local hospital and ask to speak to a psychiatrist.

Many people who are not at significant risk for HIV infection have nonetheless become anxious about AIDS. Learning the facts about HIV infection and practicing risk reduction may reduce your anxiety. If your psychological symptoms persist, consider the possibility that they may be the result of other emotional conflicts. You may benefit from psychological counseling.

6

Insurance

There are three kinds of insurance you should know about: health insurance, life insurance, and disability insurance (which provides money to live on if you are unable to work due to illness).

HEALTH INSURANCE

If you are infected with HIV, it is crucial for you to have adequate health insurance. Paying for medical care without insurance is almost prohibitively expensive. If you are forced to rely on government-funded health insurance (Medicaid), you are likely to get second-class care. If possible, plan your health insurance carefully: do not let your health insurance lapse at any time. In almost all states, it is difficult to obtain health insurance after a diagnosis of AIDS. However, in some states health insurance is available under mandated programs (risk pools and open enrollment).

The insurance industry is regulated on a state-by-state basis, and regulations and laws change frequently. Familiarize yourself with the regulations in your home state. Learn any new regulations or industry practices before buying or changing insurance policies. Ask your local AIDS service organization for advice. It is sometimes difficult to get accurate information from insurance companies—you may want to check the information they provide against that available through your state insurance commission.

Many people who receive insurance through their jobs work for companies that are self-insured, that is, medical insurance is funded by the company itself, even when administered by an insurance company. These programs are officially considered employee-benefit plans, rather than insurance policies. For this reason, they are exempt from almost all state regulations regarding insurance, and individuals lack the protection of state insurance regulations. Instead, their operation is governed by ERISA (the Employee Retirement Income Security Act of 1974). ERISA has few substantive rules about insurance. In 1974, only 5% of employees with medical insurance worked for self-insured companies. As of 1989, a majority of employees work for self-insured companies.

Employment-Based Group Insurance

Group Insurance

The easiest and best way for you to obtain insurance is through your place of employment. At many jobs you are entitled to get group health insurance, often partially financed as a component of your job's compensation. Any company with fifteen or more employees must provide group health insurance. Group health insurance is often fairly comprehensive and affordable.

Group health insurance is provided by the company for which you work itself or sold to the company by commercial insurance companies, HMOs (health maintenance organizations, described below) or Blue Cross/Blue Shield. Blue Cross/Blue Shield is a group of mostly not-for-profit insurers who offer different plans in different regions of the country.

At companies with at least twenty-five employees, insurance policies usually do not refuse to cover you because you have a medical problem; no "proof of insurability" is required. However, there may be a six- to twelve-month waiting period before you are eligible to get benefits for preexisting conditions—such as any HIV-related disorder you had before the effective date of the policy. During this time your insurance will not pay for treatment of the preexisting condition.

Small Group Insurance

Most people who work for companies with a thousand or more employees have group health insurance (85%, according to a 1989 study). However, in firms that employ less than twenty-five people, only 40% have group health coverage. Small companies cannot afford to self-insure. In order to avoid high costs, small companies often refuse to offer employees any health insurance. According to a 1987 study, two-thirds of working people without medical insurance work for firms with fewer than twenty-five employees. However, recent insurance reforms in a number of states (including New York, New Jersey, California, and Florida) require insurance companies to sell insurance to all small groups.

Small group plans are sometimes available through social or professional groups. If you are not employed, or if your employment does not offer health insurance benefits, then you should investigate joining a social group or professional organization that offers a group insurance plan. Such plans are increasingly rare, tend to be more expensive than employment-based group insurance, and are likely to get still more expensive as time goes by.

Individual Insurance

Individual health insurance (also referred to as direct-pay or nongroup insurance) is extremely expensive. Commercial insurance companies in most states are not required to write policies for people who have an increased chance of falling ill. Consequently, they will refuse you insurance coverage if they think you are at high risk for developing AIDS. For this purpose, insurance companies have the legal right to require HIV antibody testing and to refuse you coverage if you are positive. In California, where HIV-antibody testing for insurance purposes is still banned, insurance companies are allowed to discriminate on the basis of CD4 cell counts and other medical indicators. In New York, commercial insurance is available to individuals with HIV, but it is expensive and does not cover many costs.

Blue Cross/Blue Shield Open Enrollment

In a few states you can obtain individual insurance through a Blue Cross/Blue Shield open enrollment program. These policies are available without medical evidence of insurability; you may purchase such a policy even if you have AIDS. However, these policies have a number of disadvantages: some coverage may be limited, there may be a waiting period between buying the insurance and being able to use it, and in some locations only basic hospitalization coverage is available. These policies are available year-round in some states and only during specified periods in other states. You can check about the availability of an open enrollment policy by calling the Blue Cross/Blue Shield office in your area and, if necessary, double-check by calling your state insurance regulatory agency. In New York, Blue Cross/Blue Shield offers a managed care (HMO) policy.

Risk Pools May Help Cover Uninsurable People

Approximately 50% of states have created risk pools through which citizens who are otherwise uninsurable can obtain health coverage, although at an increased premium (typically about 150% of the median insurance rates). The cost of risk-pool insurance is quite high for the level of coverage provided. Few states provide assistance for those who cannot afford the high cost. In a number of states, Medicaid will help individuals pay for the cost of health insurance obtained before the disability.

Levels of Coverage

Whether you have group or individual insurance, you should read the provisions of your policy carefully. There are two basic types of health insurance: hospitalization, which pays for hospital expenses other than doctors' bills; and basic medical/major medical, which pays for some or all of doctors' fees both in and out of the hospital. Policies typically cover 60% to 80% of medical bills. Some policies have yearly or lifetime limits on reimbursement.

You may have the option of choosing different levels of coverage. If you are HIV-infected and have an increased likelihood of becoming ill, you should choose the highest level of coverage you can afford. Some policies offer coverage for other important medical expenses: home care, which allows people with AIDS to be cared for outside of the hospital, hospice care, and medications. For a higher premium, some policies offer a higher rate of reimbursement for expenses and coverage for more days per year of hospitalization. Again, buy the most coverage you can afford.

Preexisting Conditions

A preexisting condition is a medical condition that existed prior to the effective date of an insurance policy. Coverage may or may not be provided for preexisting conditions under the terms of a particular policy. Some policies cover all illnesses, whether or not they are preexisting conditions. Other policies will never pay for any preexisting condition. Still other policies pay claims relating to preexisting conditions after a specified waiting time, often eleven months from the effective date of the policy. Definitions of preexisting conditions vary widely.

Carefully review the terms of your policy that relate to preexisting conditions. If you develop AIDS, your insurer may try to claim that, because there is typically a long lag between infection with HIV and emergence of AIDS, your illness is a preexisting condition and consequently refuse to pay for your HIV-related claims. A number of such cases are now being decided. In many states, the reform of insurance regulations allow individuals "portability" of insurance. That is, a person can move from one policy to another without having to go through a new preexisting-condition period.

Continuation and Conversion of Employment-Based Coverage

If you leave your job, you can maintain your health insurance at least temporarily. Under the federal Consolidated Omnibus Budget Reconciliation Act of 1985 (COBRA), if you work for an employer with at least twenty employees, you are entitled to continue your group insurance for eighteen months after you leave your job. If the Social Security Administration determines that you are disabled at the time you leave your job, you are entitled to continue for twenty-nine months. If you change jobs, you may use COBRA to maintain your old group coverage during the waiting period before preexisting conditions are covered under the group insurance at your new job.

If you are not eligible for COBRA (because your company has fewer than twenty employees) or if your COBRA coverage runs out, you may be eligible for a conversion policy. Conversion policies convert group policies to individual policies. These individual policies usually cost more and cover much less than the group insurance. The majority of states have laws requiring companies to offer conversion policies to individuals when their COBRA coverage runs out. *To take advantage of continuation or conversion options, you must take action to change your policy immediately (often within twenty days) after leaving your job, so act promptly.* Many states have similar laws.

HMOs

Health maintenance organizations (HMOs) provide comprehensive services for a fixed, prepaid amount that is independent of the number of services actually used. If you belong to an HMO, you are only covered for treatment by those doctors who work for the HMO. The advantage of HMOs is that they pay for 100% of medical expenses and are often a good bargain financially. The (very significant) disadvantages are that there may be few or no doctors expert in treatment of HIV-related illnesses affiliated with your HMO, and you will have a limited choice of hospitals to which you can be admitted. Despite these disadvantages, individuals are increasingly being pushed into HMO plans. If you are part of an HMO, consider joining or organizing other consumers in the HMO to lobby for inclusion of HIV-expert physicians on the roster of approved doctors.

Some managed-care programs are called point-of-service plans. These plans allow the member to seek care outside the circle of approved providers and receive some reimbursement.

Limited Options for Those without Coverage

If you are diagnosed with AIDS or other HIV-related symptoms and have no health insurance, your options are:

- Get a job that will entitle you to join a group health insurance plan.
- Buy open-enrollment insurance through Blue Cross/Blue Shield if it is offered in your state and you can afford it.
- Buy risk-pool insurance if it is offered in your state and you can afford it.

- If you are under nineteen years old (or in some cases under twenty-three and single), you may be able to continue on your parents' policy and later convert this to an individual policy under your own name.
- If you are older, you may be able to move in with a family member who is able to include you under his or her health insurance coverage. This is rarely possible.
- Go on Medicaid or Medicare (government-funded health insurance) or, if you are eligible, get care through the Veterans Administration (VA).

Medicaid and the VA are the least attractive options. Medicaid (MediCal in California) is funded by federal, state, and local government. Medicaid is means-tested: if you are uninsured but have some savings, you will have to "spend down" your savings to a low level before you are eligible for Medicaid. Many private doctors do not accept Medicaid patients at all. Any people who spent time in the armed services and received an honorable discharge are eligible for medical care for AIDS through the VA. However, this care is usually not of the best quality.

Medicare is federally funded. There is a two-year waiting period from the time of diagnosis before a person with AIDS becomes eligible for Medicare, and even then Medicare does not cover all your bills. It does not cover medication. For more information about Medicare and Medicaid, contact a social worker or a caseworker from an AIDS service organization.

Insurance May Not Cover All Costs

Thirty-five to thirty-seven million U.S. citizens have no health insurance and are not receiving Medicaid. Even if you do have health insurance, you may still have difficulty meeting medical expenses if you develop AIDS. Policies usually require that you pay some minimum amount per year (called the deductible) before insurance will pay anything. Also "coinsurance" means that you may have to pay a fixed percentage (typically 20%) of your bills even after you meet the deductible. Policies may have a limit on benefits paid per hospital stay or a lifetime cap on benefits. If your costs exceed the maximum, you will have to pay the difference. Also, many policies do not reimburse for medication, hospice, or home-care costs. Finally, you should be aware that most policies will not reimburse you for nonprescription treatments.

There is general agreement on the need for reform, and for a period of time, it appeared that a more equitable system might be established. Efforts at this have so far failed. In the current political times the outlook is bleak, and the situation may even worsen for many individuals.

LIFE INSURANCE

Many people who are HIV-infected or have AIDS wish to obtain life insurance to protect their life partners or dependents. Virtually all insurance companies require applicants for policies of $100,000 or more to be HIV antibody tested. Applicants testing positive for HIV antibody are rejected. Also, insurers have resisted paying benefits on policies where the policyholder died of AIDS, often claiming that the policyholder misrepresented his or her state of health when the insurance was purchased. Contact a sympathetic insurance agent who is knowledgeable about HIV disease for more information.

Life insurance is useful to people living with AIDS because it is possible to sell your life insurance policy to obtain money to live on if you are sick. Policies are bought by companies referred to as viatical settlement companies. They pay you money in return for naming them as the beneficiary of the life insurance policy.

It is important to get knowledgeable advice about viatical settlements. The federal government may consider such a settlement to be taxable income. If you are on Medicaid, receiving a settlement may raise your income level and jeopardize your Medicaid eligibility.

The viatical settlement business is beginning to be regulated and licensed. It is best to choose a licensed company.

Some life insurance companies will themselves make settlements for individuals. This is referred to as accelerated benefits and often provides a better return than viatical settlements.

REPLACING INCOME LOST DURING ILLNESS

If you become ill and are unable to work, you will need another source of income. Short-term disability insurance (usually six months) is commonly provided through employers. Some jobs also provide long-term disability insurance that will pay a significant portion of your former earnings. These policies can also be purchased privately. Again, it is crucial to investigate possibilities before you become ill.

There are a number of government-sponsored income-replacement programs. Entitlement programs vary from state to state and city to city. Go to a local AIDS organization or hospital social worker for help in obtaining these benefits. The benefits and entitlements system can be bewilderingly complex: you will definitely need help threading your way through the maze.

Federal Programs

Try to get either federal disability insurance or supplemental security income through the Social Security Administration. If you cannot work because of AIDS, you are probably entitled to one of these two benefits. The Social Security Administration decides whether people in this situation are disabled on a case-by-case basis. Be prepared to face a lot of red tape.

Other Programs

State disability programs may pay benefits if you cannot work at your customary occupation but are capable of other work. Other programs you may be eligible for are food stamp programs (administered by your local government) and veterans benefit programs (administered by the Veterans Administration). You may also be eligible for local public assistance or welfare benefits. Some communities have private or publicly funded programs that provide special assistance for people with AIDS, such as help for the homebound, meal delivery service, and financial aid for expensive medications such as AZT (see the Resource Guide).

7

Discrimination and Confidentiality

Harassment and discrimination against people who have or are perceived to have HIV infection or AIDS has become a serious problem nationwide. People with AIDS have lost jobs and housing and face ostracism because of bias and irrational fear of contagion. Reports of violence against gay men and lesbians have increased dramatically in recent years.[1] Discrimination against people with AIDS or HIV infection is illegal in most situations, but enforcement can be difficult. Guarding your civil rights takes knowledge and effort.

Get legal help if you are faced with harassment or discrimination, as redress is sometimes available. The laws surrounding discrimination are complicated, changing, and vary depending on whether federal, state, or local law is involved. File complaints *quickly*, since laws may invalidate complaints filed too long after the offending action—this means you may have to act within a few weeks of the date of any incident. In most cases, it is useful to contact a government agency to get help. Call the U.S. Health and Human Services Office of Civil Rights to get information about a branch near you. You can also call your state or city office of human or civil rights.

Although occasional complaints are settled rapidly, most take years to complete. The benefit of such action may not be to the individual involved but may help to prevent future discrimination against others. Only a brief summary of some important points can be given here. The Resource Guide lists sources of more detailed information.

Patterns of Discrimination

The American Civil Liberties Union (ACLU) AIDS Project conducted a survey of state and civil rights agencies concerning HIV discrimination. From 1983 to 1988, 260 agencies reported about 13,000 complaints of HIV discrimination. Of these complaints:

- 37% were related to employment.
- 13% were related to insurance.
- 10% were related to government service programs (e.g., delays and obstacles in Medicaid and other funding, discriminatory treatment of prisoners).
- 16% were related to housing.
- 16% were related to public accommodation (theaters, restaurants, barbers, libraries, gymnasiums, swimming pools, medical offices, shops, etc.), most often denial of services by dentists and nursing homes.
- 5% were related to health care.

EMPLOYMENT, HOUSING, AND SCHOOLING

The primary source of protection against discrimination for people with AIDS is the Americans with Disabilities Act (ADA), which was passed by the U.S. Congress in 1990. The ADA prohibits discrimination against those with disabilities, including HIV disease. This bill took full effect four years after passage. ADA also extends to the disabled the enforcement provisions under Title VI of the Civil Rights Act of 1964 (including injunctive relief and back pay). Prior to the enactment of the ADA, HIV discrimination was largely illegal federally under section 504 of the United States Rehabilitation Act. However, this act applied only to institutions that received federal funding. This act and a number of other federal and state antidiscrimination measures are still in force and cover areas not dealt with by the ADA.

Employment Discrimination

HIV antibody testing is not permitted in an employment setting, since the use of tests to screen out disabled persons is prohibited by the Rehabilitation Act. Most states have laws prohibiting discrimination against the disabled in employment, and many states have recently strengthened these laws. Laws are different in each state: some cover only public employees or employees of organizations with more than sixteen workers; some exclude those with communicable diseases; and some exclude those who are only *perceived* as disabled (that is, thought by others to be disabled). The ADA mandates reasonable accommodation for the disabled in employment settings. "Reasonable accommodation" is defined as altering the job conditions or the physical setting of the job so that a disabled individual who can perform the essential central functions of a job can do the work. Such accommodations must not cause "undue hardship" to the employee. The ADA provides guidance about the applicability and scope of reasonable accommodation.

If you are a union member, your collective bargaining agreement may provide additional protection because it places limits on the arbitrary dismissal of an employee.

Discrimination in Housing

The eviction of people thought to have AIDS and the refusal to sell homes to such people are common housing problems. The Federal Fair Housing Act provides protection against discrimination in housing for all disabled people, including those with HIV disease. Most states have laws protecting disabled people that may provide protection in cases of housing discrimination against people with AIDS or HIV infection. Some states and municipalities have passed ordinances prohibiting housing discrimination against people who have or are perceived to have AIDS or HIV infection.

Discrimination in Schools

The federal Centers for Disease Control (CDC) says that school-age children with AIDS should be allowed to attend school.[2] The National Association of State Boards of Education has developed a set of guidelines regarding HIV infection in the school setting.[3] These guidelines declare that any HIV-infected students, teachers, and school staff members able to attend class or work should not suffer exclusion or discrimination. The only exception is when the HIV-infected adult or child has a secondary contagious disease such as tuberculosis that would warrant action under existing public health laws.

Protection for children denied access to schooling may be found in the ADA, section 504 of the Rehabilitation Act, in the Federal Education for All Handicapped Children Act, and under state and local law.

Despite this, in the 1980s there were many instances of discrimination in the education of children with HIV. This controversy seems to have lessened since the late 1980s.

Discrimination Against HIV-Infected Health Care Workers

Despite overwhelming scientific evidence that HIV is not transmitted from health care workers to patients, a number of health care workers have been transferred to non-patient-contact duties or have been fired. Unfortunately, courts have taken an unscientific position and generally upheld this discrimination.

Barriers to Fighting Discrimination

Despite legislation protecting people with AIDS against a wide variety of forms of discrimination, AIDS-related discrimination continues. People with AIDS have difficulty finding knowledgeable lawyers willing to represent them, and difficulty having their cases handled quickly enough to be of any benefit.[4] Fear of stigmatization, retribution, and the difficulty of pursuing legal redress discourage many who are discriminated against from taking action. According to the ACLU, communities of color are even more underrepresented than others with HIV disease in getting access to protection against discrimination.

GOVERNMENTAL POLICIES AFFECTING PEOPLE WITH AIDS AND HIV INFECTION

Employment

The federal government requires all applicants for employment or service in certain programs to take the HIV antibody test. These include the Peace Corps, the Foreign Service of the State Department, the armed forces, the state National Guard, and residential training programs of the Job Corps. Discrimination is practiced against those who test positive. Applicants for the Peace Corps and the Foreign Service who test positive are rejected. Current members of the Foreign Service who are positive or have spouses or dependent children who test positive are barred from most posts outside the United States. Job Corps students are subjected to repeated psychological tests that the government claims can establish whether an individual is likely to act to transmit HIV to others.

Military Service

All military and National Guard personnel and all recruits are subjected to HIV antibody testing. Army recruits, ROTC students, service academy cadets, and all candidates for officer service are punished with expulsion if they are found to be infected with HIV. Active-duty personnel who test positive are not expelled, but are subject to involuntary change and limitation of duties, often without rational justification. Their confidentiality is sometimes violated, causing rumor and harassment. Also, HIV-infected soldiers are subject to court-martial and punitive discharge unless they comply with military guidelines to prevent HIV transmission—guidelines that can be unreasonably restrictive when compared with public health recommendations promulgated by other branches of the government. If you are diagnosed with AIDS while you are in the military, get legal help *immediately.*

An amendment under consideration by Congress in 1995 (the Dornan amendment) may mandate discharge for every HIV-infected person in the military. Discharge would be honorable, but would nonetheless damage careers and lives and cost the government unnecessary dollars.

In general, there is no patient-doctor confidentiality in the military. Information a military patient tells his or her military doctor may, with some limits, be used in court-martial proceedings. The military often prolongs review by medical and physical evaluation boards that must precede disability retirement and payment of benefits, with the effect that personnel sick with AIDS may die without getting the care or benefits to which their military service entitled them.

Immigration

Since December 1987, all applicants for citizenship and resident alien status ("green card") and for amnesty and refugee status have been obliged to be HIV antibody tested and, if positive, are (with rare exceptions) excluded. If you have already gained citizenship or resident alien status, you are not required to be tested.

According to law, short-term travelers to the United States may also be excluded if they are found out to be

HIV-positive. However, this regulation is rarely put into practice. Initially, this was mandated through the so-called Helms Amendment. However, this law was repealed in 1990 and was replaced by the immigration act of 1990, which created a list of excludable diseases on the basis of danger to public health. The secretary of health and human services, backed by the country's public health organizations, recommended that only infectious tuberculosis be a basis for exclusion. However, the U.S. Justice Department ignored this recommendation and ordered that HIV disease be restored to the list. As of 1991, the government has, in practice, allowed HIV-infected people to enter the country temporarily but tests would-be immigrants and excludes those who are HIV-infected.

Prisoners

A large number of HIV-infected Americans are incarcerated in federal, state, and local prisons. Medical care in prison systems is poor: it is almost impossible for an HIV-infected prisoner to get the sophisticated medical care that HIV-related illness requires. Studies have shown that prisoners with AIDS have a shorter life span than nonprisoners with AIDS. The U.S. Supreme Court has ruled that prisoners have a constitutional right to adequate health care.[5] In some cases, prisoners have been able to obtain legal assistance to improve the quality of health care they receive.

As of 1991, the Federal Bureau of Prisons and a number of state prison systems mandate HIV antibody testing. Some prisons segregate prisoners with HIV infection or AIDS, often in facilities with even worse conditions than those suffered by the general prison population. Despite the fact that drug use and sexual activity between male prisoners is commonplace, most prisons do not make sterile injection equipment or condoms available to prisoners. Counseling and AIDS education for prisoners and corrections officers has been inadequate. Possible sources of advice for prisoners are listed in the Resource Guide. Prisoners may also be able to obtain help from local AIDS service organizations.

CONFIDENTIALITY

If you have AIDS or HIV infection, keep this information secret from all branches of the government, organizations, employers, or individuals who might discriminate against you—except as required to obtain medical care or funds such as insurance reimbursements or disability payments. The laws and regulations governing confidentiality of medical records are complicated, different in each state, and changing. It is best to be HIV antibody tested anonymously.

Reporting of AIDS or HIV Infection

All states require that physicians report the identities of individuals diagnosed with AIDS to either state or local health authorities. Physicians have been required to report other communicable and sexually transmissible diseases for a number of years. Public health authorities have a good record of maintaining the confidentiality of such information. Information about the identities of people newly diagnosed with AIDS is used to help track the progress of the epidemic.

Physician-Patient Confidentiality

Make sure your physician knows that you are extremely concerned about confidentiality. Physicians are bound by two principles that may at times be contradictory: the *duty to maintain confidentiality* and the *duty to warn.* The duty to warn might be construed to require a physician to inform others potentially at risk, such as sexual partners of people who are HIV-infected. Recent legal trends allow physicians broader discretion in disclosing HIV status while protecting them from punishment for failure to disclose.

Most state laws permit disclosure without consent to public health officials to comply with public health laws. In addition some states allow disclosure of positive HIV status to certain specified individuals including health care workers providing treatment, funeral personnel, and sexual and needle-sharing partners. Your physician may have the right to notify your sexual partners without your consent but without disclosing your identity. Check with your local AIDS organization for the laws that apply in your state. If you discover that you are infected with HIV, you may want to consider informing past sexual partners of this fact yourself, especially if they are unlikely to think that they may have been exposed to the virus.

Health care providers cannot release information from your medical chart without your explicit written consent. At times you may have to sign a written consent to release information: for example, if your insurance company requires information before reimbursing you for medical expenses. If this situation arises, discuss with your doctor exactly what information will be released.

Hospitals

You may face breaches of confidentiality in medical settings, particularly hospitals. When you are hospitalized, many people have access to your medical chart. Knowledge of an AIDS diagnosis or an HIV infection is supposed to be limited to members of the "treatment team" *only*, who need the information in order to care for you properly. Hospital personnel do not need to know whether you are HIV-infected or have AIDS in order to protect themselves: standard infection-control procedures—which should be followed at all times with all patients—should be adequate. However, confidentiality is not well protected in hospitals.

Some hospitals routinely screen patients for HIV antibody, but you should always "opt out" and refuse to be HIV antibody tested in a hospital setting unless testing is clinically indicated for diagnostic purposes in your particular case. If you are a subject in an AIDS research study, ask if explicit written provisions have been made to protect your confidentiality.

Employee Clinics

Clinics maintained by an employer do not offer adequate protection for your confidentiality. The same may be true of clinics maintained by unions. Do not allow yourself to be HIV antibody tested in such a clinic, unless the testing is anonymous. Think carefully about the benefits and costs of telling any physician in such a clinic that you have tested antibody positive. If your employer or clinic physician insists that you must be HIV antibody tested, you may sue them under ADA Section 504 of the Federal Rehabilitation Act and relevant state and local legislation.

Courtroom Proceedings

HIV-infected people held in custody pending jury trial are suffering unequal treatment in many courtrooms across the nation. Sometimes, officers of the court and the correctional system have worn "protective" devices such as rubber gloves or surgical masks, incorrectly believing they are in danger of becoming HIV-infected through their contact with the defendant. This is medically unnecessary, reveals the defendant's infected status to the courtroom, violates confidentiality, and may prejudice a defendant's case by influencing a jury or a judge.

TRAVEL TO FOREIGN COUNTRIES

Over fifty countries now place some travel restrictions on HIV-infected people. These restrictions primarily apply to those visitors who are planning long-term stays, such as students or migrant workers. Permanent immigration of HIV-infected people is probably barred by almost all countries.

The regulations vary widely. Check with the embassy of foreign countries you plan to visit to get up-to-the-minute information about their requirements. A legal scholar states, "Restrictions based upon HIV infection . . . are unjustifiable and may be counterproductive to the control of HIV transmission. Moreover, they are likely to jeopardize prevention efforts."[6]

RESOURCE GUIDE

National AIDS Information Hot Line
U.S. Public Health Service

English	(800) 342-2437
Español	(800) 344-7432
Hearing-impaired/TDD	(800) 243-7889

Local AIDS Organizations and Hot Lines

These organizations can give you information about HIV services in your area, including anonymous HIV antibody testing and medical treatment.

State and City		Organization	Telephone Number
AZ	Phoenix	Arizona AIDS Project	(602) 265-3300
CA	Los Angeles	AIDS Project/L.A.	(213) 876-2437
CA	Los Angeles	AIDS Project/L.A. (So. Cal.)	(213) 993-1600
CA	San Francisco	San Francisco AIDS Foundation	(415) 863-2437
CA	San Francisco	San Francisco AIDS Foundation	(800) 367-2437
CO	Denver	Colorado AIDS Project	(303) 837-0166
DC	Washington	DC AIDS Information Line (Whitman Walker)	(202) 332-2437
FL	Miami	Health Crisis Network	(305) 751-7751
GA	Atlanta	Georgia AIDS Information Line	(404) 876-9944
IL	Chicago	AIDS Hotline	(800) 243-2437
LA	New Orleans	New Orleans AIDS Task Force	(504) 944-2437
LA	New Orleans	New Orleans AIDS Task Force (LA)	(800) 992-4379

State and City		Organization	Telephone Number
MA	Boston	AIDS Action Committee of Massachusetts	(617) 536-7733
MD	Baltimore	Maryland AIDS Hotline	(800) 638-6252
MI	Royal Oak	Wellness Networks (MI)	(800) 872-2437
MN	Minneapolis	Minnesota AIDS Hotline	(800) 248-2437
MO	St. Louis	St. Louis Effort for AIDS	(314) 367-2382
NJ	New Jersey	Hyacinth Foundation Hotline	(800) 433-0254
NJ	New Jersey	New Jersey AIDS Foundation	(201) 246-0204
NY	New York City	Gay Men's Health Crisis	(212) 807-6655
NY	New York City	People With AIDS Coalition	(212) 647-1415
OH	Columbus	Columbus AIDS Task Force	(614) 488-2437
PA	Philadelphia	PCHA Hotline	(215) 985-2437
PR	San Juan	Puerto Rico AIDS Foundation	(809) 782-9600
TX	Dallas	Oaklawn AIDS Project Infoline	(800) 299-2437
TX	Houston	AIDS Foundation Houston Hotline	(713) 524-2437
WA	Seattle	Northwest AIDS Foundation	(206) 329-6923
WI	Milwaukee	Milwaukee AIDS Project (WI)	(800) 334-2437
WI	Milwaukee	Milwaukee AIDS Project	(414) 273-2437

HIV-2 Testing

For anonymous HIV-2 testing, have your physician contact: CDC, AIDS Program, Laboratory Investigation Branch (404) 639-3174

Treatment Guides

The numbers listed are for reliable free or low-cost periodicals about treatment, including experimental drugs.

AIDS/HIV Treatment Directory (American Foundation for AIDS Research)	(800) 458-5231
AIDS Treatment News (John James)	(415) 255-0588
Treatment Issues (GMHC)	(212) 337-3505
PI Perspectives (Project Inform), national number	(800) 822-7422
From California	(800) 334-7422
Beta	(415) 863-2437

Financial Assistance for HIV Drugs

Information on the AIDS Drug Reimbursement Program is
generally available by calling the department of health in
your county. Some direct sources of information are:

Federal

Richard Schulman
Health Resources and Services Administration, AIDS
Drug Reimbursement Program   (301) 443-4170

NY State AIDS Drug Assistance Program
    (ADAP)   (800) 542-2437

CA State Office of AIDS   (916) 324-8429

Treatment Information Hot Lines

To get information about clinical trials in your area that
are open for enrollment, call 800-TRIALS-A (800-874-
2572). Call Monday through Friday, 9 A.M. to 7 P.M., EST.
This is an information service sponsored by the Centers for
Disease Control (CDC). Information is available in both
Spanish and English. You will get to speak to someone in
person who will give you information about government-
approved clinical trials and also about specific drugs, both
antivirals and those for opportunistic infections. They will
do computer searches for you. Services are free. For information about new drug studies being done at the National
Institutes of Health, call (800) 243-7644. For information
about FDA-approved treatments for HIV, call the federal
AIDS Treatment Information Service at (800) 448-0440.

Buyers' Groups

Two reliable buyers' clubs (groups that supply "under-
ground" AIDS drugs) are:

| People With AIDS Health Group | (212) 255-0520 |
| Healing Alternatives Foundation | (415) 626-2316 |

Call these two clubs for information about the reliability of buyers' clubs in your area.

Other Groups That Provide HIV-Related Services

Sexual minorities (gay men and lesbians)

Lambda Legal Defense and Education Fund	(212) 995-8585
National Gay and Lesbian Task Force (NGLTF)	(202) 332-6483
	(415) 563-0724
Human Rights Campaign Fund (HRCF)	(202) 628-4160
ACT UP/NY	(212) 564-2437
NY Lesbian & Gay Anti-Violence Project, AIDS-Related Crime Hot Line	(212) 807-0197
NY Gay & Lesbian Community Center	(212) 620-7310
LA Gay & Lesbian Community Center	(213) 993-7400
TAG (Treatment Action Group)	(212) 260-0300

Women

Women's AIDS Network (SF AIDS Foundation)	(415) 864-5855 ext. 2007
Planned Parenthood	NY (212) 541-7800
	SF (415) 441-7858

Ethnic and racial minorities

National Minority AIDS Council	(202) 544-1076
IMPACT	(202) 546-7228
National Council La Raza—AIDS Project	(202) 785-1670
Midwest Hispanic AIDS Coalition	(312) 772-8195
COSSMHO (Hispanic health group)	(202) 387-5000
People of Color Against AIDS Network (Washington State)	(206) 322-7061

Hemophiliacs

National Hemophilia Foundation   (212) 219-8180

Substance users (narcotics, alcohol, etc.)

ADAPT (Association for Drug Abuse
    Prevention and Treatment)   (718) 665-5421
Alcoholics Anonymous Intergroup   NY (212) 647-1680
                                           SF (415) 621-1326
                                           LA (213) 936-4343

Children/parents

Pediatric AIDS Foundation   (310) 395-9051

Teenagers

Hetrick-Martin Institute for Protection of
    Lesbian and Gay Youth   (212) 941-9555

Health Insurance

For information about insurance matters, contact your
local AIDS organization or your state insurance commission. Many insurers pool underwriting reports on their
applicants and policyholders through a clearinghouse
called MIB. Most of the information in MIB files refers to
medical history, but such subjects as drug abuse, sexual
orientation, and general "lifestyle" issues are also included.
You can challenge information you think is incorrect. MIB
will send a copy of your file to your physician if you write to
MIB, P.O. Box 105, Essex Station, Boston, MA 02112.

Legal Matters

American Civil Liberties Union—Lesbian   (212) 944-9800
    and Gay Rights Project   ext. 545
National Lawyers Guild AIDS Network   (415) 285-5066
Intergovernmental Health Policy
    Project—AIDS Policy Center (George
    Washington University)   (202) 872-1445

Military

Military Law Task Force (National
    Military Project on AIDS)   (619) 233-1701
Citizen Soldier   (212) 777-3470
Midwest Committee for Military
    Counseling   (312) 939-3349
CCCO   (415) 474-3002
    (215) 545-4626

Immigration

The Center for Immigrants' Rights   (212) 505-6890
National Network for Immigrants' and
    Refugee Rights   (510) 465-1984

Prisoners

American Civil Liberties Union National
    Prison Project   (202) 544-1681

Information Resources for Travelers

Call the Centers for Disease Control (CDC) International Travelers Hot Line at (404) 332-4555 for up-to-date health information for travelers, including current areas of infectious disease and current vaccination requirements for travel to various countries.

A booklet is also available from the CDC entitled "Health Information for International Travel" ($5). Call (202) 783-3238.

NOTES

AIM—Annals of Internal Medicine
JAMA—Journal of the American Medical Association
MMWR—Morbidity and Mortality Weekly Report
NEJM—New England Journal of Medicine

Chapter 1

1. CDC, *HIV/AIDS Surveillance Report*, 7, no. 1 (1995): 5.
2. World Health Organization, "The HIV/AIDS Pandemic: 1994 overview," WHO/GPA/TCO/SEF/94.4.
3. J. L. Jones et al., "Surveillance of AIDS-Defining Conditions in the United States Adult/Adolescent Spectrum of HIV Disease Project Group," *AIDS* 8, no. 10 (October 1994): 1489–93.
4. J. Nelson et al., "Human immunodeficiency virus detected in bowel epithelium from patients with gastrointestinal symptoms," *Lancet* I:8580 (February 6, 1988): 259–62.
5. R. Pomerantz et al., "Infection of the retina by human immunodeficiency virus type I," *NEJM* 317, no. 26: 1643–47.
6. G. Elder and J. Sever, "Neurologic disorders associated with AIDS retroviral infection," *Review of Infectious Diseases* 10, no. 2 (March–April 1988): 286–302.
7. CDC, *HIV/AIDS Surveillance Report*, 1.
8. H. Libman et al., *"HIV Infection: A Clinical Manual"* (Boston: Little, Brown, and Company, 1993), 12.
9. A. Glatt, et al., "Treatment of infections associated with human immunodeficiency virus," *NEJM* 318, no. 22 (June 22, 1988): 1439–48.

10. M. Marco et al., "The KS Project Report: current issues in research and treatment of Kaposi's sarcoma" (Treatment Action Group, 1994).

11. D. Kotler, "Practical Evaluation of Fever and Wasting" (AMFAR conference: Management of the HIV-Infected Patient, March 31–April 2, 1995).

12. M. A. Bacellar et al., "Temporal trends in the incidence of HIV-1-related neurologic diseases: Multicenter AIDS Cohort Study, 1985–1992," *Neurology* 44 (1994): 1892–1900.

13. I. Grant et al., "Evidence for early central nervous system involvement in the acquired immunodeficiency syndrome (AIDS) and other human immunodeficiency virus (HIV) infections," *AIM* 107, no. 6 (December 1987): 828–36.

14. Elder and Sever, "Neurologic disorders," 286–302.

15. O. Selnes et al., "Longitudinal neuropsychological (NP) evaluation of healthy HIV-1 infected homosexual men: the Multicenter AIDS Cohort Study (MACS) [abstract]" (4th International Conference on AIDS, Stockholm, June 12–16, 1988), 2:8561.

16. J. McArthur, "Neurological Diseases Associated with Human Immunodeficiency Virus Type 1 Infection," *Current Therapy in Neurological Disease*, 146.

17. P. Hopewell et al. in M. Sande et al., *The Medical Management of AIDS*, 4th ed. (1995), chap. 20.

18. C. Boucher et al., "HIV-1 biological phenotype and the development of zidovudine resistance in relation to disease progression in asymptomatic individuals during treatment," *AIDS* 6 (1992): 1259–64.

19. Libman et al., "HIV Infection," 233–62.

20. M. Fischl in M. Sande et al., *The Medical Management of AIDS*, 4th ed. (Philadelphia: W.B. Saunders Company, 1995), 141–60.

21. A. Lifson, "Do alternative modes of transmission of human immunodeficiency virus exist? *JAMA* 259, no. 9 (March 4, 1988): 1353.

22. CDC, "Recommendations for preventing transmission of infection with HTLV-III/LAV in the workplace," *MMWR* 34 (1985): 681–86, 691–95.

23. Pomerantz et al., "Infection of the retina," 1643–47.

24. J. Pudney et al., "Pre-ejaculatory fluid as a potential

vector for sexual transmission of HIV-1," *Lancet* 340 (December 1992): 1470.

25. G. Ilaria, "Detection of HIV-1 DNA sequences in preejaculatory fluid [letter]," *Lancet* 340 (8833) (December 1992): 1469.

26. G. Friedland and R. Klein, "Transmission of the human immunodeficiency virus," *NEJM* 317, no. 18 (October 1987): 1125–35.

27. M. Vogt et al., "Isolation patterns of the human immunodeficiency virus from cervical secretions during the menstrual cycle of women at risk for the acquired immunodeficiency syndrome," *AIM* 106, no. 3 (March 1987): 380–82.

28. M. R. Rabinovitch, J. M. Iversen, and L. Resnick, "Anti-infectivity activity of human salivary secretions towards human immunodeficiency virus," *Crit. Rev. Oral. Biol. Med.* 4, no. 3–4 (1993): 455–59.

29. Institute of Medicine, National Academy of Sciences, *Confronting AIDS* (1986), 98.

30. D. Ho et al., "Infrequency of isolation of HTLV-III virus from saliva in AIDS," *NEJM* 313 (1985): 1606.

31. CDC, "Acquired immunodeficiency syndrome (AIDS) in Western Palm Beach County, Florida," *MMWR* 35 (1986): 609–12.

32. A. Zuckerman, "AIDS and insects," *British Medical Journal* 292 (1986): 1094–95.

33. L. Martin et al., "Disinfection and inactivation of human T-lymphotropic virus type III/lymphadenopathy-associated virus," *Journal of Infectious Diseases* 152 (1985): 400–403.

34. Institute of Medicine, National Academy of Sciences, *Confronting AIDS* (1986), 10.

35. G. Friedland et al., "Lack of transmission of HTLV-III/LAV infection to household contacts of patients with AIDS," *NEJM* 314 (1986): 344–49.

36. Friedland and Klein, "Transmission of the human immunodeficiency virus," 1125–35.

37. T. Peterman, "Risk of HTLV-III/LAV transmission to household contacts of persons with transfusion-associated HTLV-III/LAV infection" (read before the 2nd International Conference on AIDS, Paris, June 23–25, 1986).

38. CDC, "Recommendations for preventing transmission of

infection with HTLV-III/LAV in the workplace," *MMWR* 34 (1985): 681–86, 691–95.

Chapter 2

1. CDC, *HIV/AIDS Surveillance Report,* 7, no. 1 (1995): 8.

2. H. Jaffe, "HIV/AIDS Epidemiology: The Past and the Future" (AMFAR conference: Management of the HIV-Infected Patient, March 31–April 2, 1995).

3. S. Chu et al., "Female-to-female sexual contact and HIV transmission," *JAMA* 272, no. 6 (1994): 433.

4. J. Buehler et al. in M. Sande et al., *The Medical Management of AIDS,* 4th ed. (Philadelphia: W.B. Saunders Company, 1995), 6.

5. Jaffe, "HIV/AIDS Epidemiology."

6. N. Padian, "Male-to-female transmission of human immunodeficiency virus," *JAMA* 258, no. 6 (August 1987): 788–90.

7. N. Padian, "Female-to-male transmission of human immunodeficiency virus," *JAMA* 266 (1991): 1664–67.

8. CDC, *HIV/AIDS Surveillance Report,* 21.

9. J. Goedert et al., "Heterosexual transmission of human immunodeficiency virus (HIV); association with severe T4-cell depletion in male hemophiliacs [abstract]" (3rd International Conference on AIDS, Washington, D.C., June 1–5, 1987), 106.

10. S. Staprans et al. in M. Sande et al., *The Medical Management of AIDS,* 4th ed. (Philadelphia: W.B. Saunders Company, 1995), 638–39.

11. T. Quinn et al., "Human immunodeficiency virus infection among patients attending clinics for sexually transmitted diseases," *NEJM* 318, no. 4 (1988): 197–203.

12. E. Telzak et al., "HIV-1 Seroconversion in Patients with and without Genital Ulcer Disease," *AIM* 119, no. 12 (December 1993): 1181–86.

13. CDC, "Human immunodeficiency virus infection in the United States: a review of current knowledge," *MMWR* 36, suppl. no. S-6 (1987): 1–46.

14. D. Des Jarlais et al., "Development of AIDS, HIV seroconversion, and cofactors for T4-cell loss in a cohort of intravenous drug users," *AIDS: An International Bimonthly* 1 (1987): 105–11.

15. CDC, *HIV/AIDS Surveillance Report,* 8.

111

16. D. Landers et al. in M. Sande et al., *The Medical Management of AIDS*, 4th ed. (Philadelphia: W.B. Saunders Company, 1995), 614.

17. "European Collaborative Study: Risk factors for mother-to-child transmission of HIV-1," *Lancet* 339 (1992): 1007–12.

18. J. Moreno et al., "Human immunodeficiency virus infection during pregnancy," *Clin. Obstet. Gynecol.* 35 (1992): 813–20.

19. M. Oxtoby, "Perinatally acquired human immunodeficiency virus infection," *Pediatric Infectious Disease Journal* 9 (1990): 606–9.

20. American College of Obstetricians and Gynecologists, "Prevention of HIV Infection and AIDS" (ACOG Committee Statement, 1987), 1–8.

21. CDC, "Recommendations for assisting in the prevention of perinatal transmission of human lymphotropic virus type III/lymphadenopathy associated virus and acquired immunodeficiency syndrome," *MMWR* 34 (1985): 681–99.

22. M. Oxtoby, "Vertically acquired HIV infection in the United States," in P. Pizzo et al., *Pediatric AIDS* (Malvern, PA: Williams & Wilkins, 1994): 2–20.

23. "European Collaborative Study," 1007–12.

24. Moreno et al., "Human immunodeficiency virus," 813–20.

25. Oxtoby, "Perinatally acquired infection," 606–9.

26. E. Connor et al., "Reduction of Maternal-Infant Transmission of Human Immunodeficiency Virus Type 1 with Zidovudine Treatment," *NEJM* 331, no. 18 (November 1994): 1173–80.

27. M. Hagen et al., "Human Immunodeficiency Virus Infection in Health Care Workers," *Arch. Intern. Med.* 149 (July 1989): 1541.

28. CDC, *HIV/AIDS Surveillance Report*, 15.

29. CDC, "Guidelines for prevention of transmission of human immunodeficiency virus and hepatitis B virus to health-care and public-safety workers," *MMWR* 38 (June 1989): 56.

30. C. Ciesielski et al., "Transmission of human immunodeficiency virus in a dental practice," *AIM* 116 (1992): 798–805.

31. CDC, *HIV/AIDS Surveillance Report*, 20.

32. CDC, "Self-reported change in sexual behaviors among homosexual and bisexual men from the San Francisco City Clinic cohort," *MMWR* 36, no. 12 (April 3, 1987): 187–89.

33. CDC, *HIV/AIDS Surveillance Report,* 8 and 12.

34. G. Lemp et al., "Seroprevalence of HIV and risk behaviors among young homosexual and bisexual men: The San Francisco/Berkeley Young Men's Survey," *JAMA* 272, no. 6 (August 1, 1994): 449–54.

35. L. Dean et al., "Rates of Unprotected Anal and Oral Sex in a Cohort of Young Gay Men in New York City," (International Conference on AIDS, 1993) (abstract no. PO-D06-3603), vol. 9 (2), 818.

36. CDC, *HIV/AIDS Surveillance Report,* 10.

37. S. Melnick, "Survival and disease progression according to gender of patients with HIV infection," *JAMA* 272 (December 1994): 1915–21.

38. CDC, *HIV/AIDS Surveillance Report,* 5, 12.

39. World Health Organization, *AIDS Surveillance Report* (update), July 1, 1990.

40. World Health Organization/Global Programme of AIDS (WHO/GPA), press release no. 53, July 1994, 3.

41. World Health Organization, *AIDS Surveillance Report.*

42. W. Johnston, *The Catastrophe Ahead* (Westport, CT: Praeger Publishers, 1990), 7.

43. R. Voelker, "Model Predicts Huge Jump in AIDS in Coming Years," *American Medical News,* December 1994.

Chapter 3

1. CDC, "Recommendations for preventing transmission of infection with HTLV-III/LAV in the workplace," *MMWR* 34 (1985): 681–86, 691–95.

2. CDC, "Guidelines for prevention of transmission of human immunodeficiency virus and hepatitis B virus to health-care and public-safety workers," *MMWR* 38 (June 23, 1989): 56.

3. CDC, "Human immunodeficiency virus infection in transfusion recipients and their family members," *MMWR* 36 (1987): 137–40.

4. D. C. Des Jarlais et al., "Development of AIDS, HIV seroconversion, and cofactors for T4-cell loss in a cohort of intravenous drug users," *AIDS: An International Bimonthly* 1 (1987): 105–11.

5. R. Hahn et al., "Prevalence of HIV infection among intravenous drug users in the United States," *JAMA* 261, no. 18 (May 12, 1989): 2677–84.

6. J. Schmalz, "Addicts to get needles in plan to curb AIDS," *The New York Times*, January 31, 1988, 1.

7. Des Jarlais et al., "Development of AIDS," 105–11.

8. Institute of Medicine, National Academy of Sciences, *Confronting AIDS* (1986), 112.

9. M. T. Schechter et al., "Can HTLV-III be transmitted orally?" *Lancet* 1 (1985): 379.

10. A. Lifson, "HIV Transmission through Specific Oral-Genital Sexual Practices," *The AIDS Reader* 4, no. 4 (July/August 1994): 129–30.

11. M. Conant et al., "Condoms prevent transmission of AIDS-associated retrovirus," *JAMA* 255 (1986): 1706.

12. D. P. Francis et al., "The prevention of acquired immunodeficiency syndrome in the United States," *JAMA* 257 (1987): 1360.

13. W. Winkelstein et al., "Sexual practices and risk of infection by the human immunodeficiency virus." *JAMA* 257, no. 3 (January 16, 1987): 321–25.

14. N. Padian, "Male-to-female transmission of human immunodeficiency virus," *JAMA* 258, no. 6 (August 14, 1987): 788–90.

15. M. Samuel, "What Does Risk Mean? Prospective and Cross-Sectional Studies, HIV Transmission through Specific Oral-Genital Sexual Practices," *The AIDS Reader* 4, no. 4 (July/August 1994): 131–32.

16. Winkelstein et al., "Sexual practices and risk," 321–25.

17. C. Riejtmeijer et al., "Condoms as physical and chemical barriers against human immunodeficiency virus," *JAMA* 259, no. 12 (March 25, 1988): 1851–53.

18. CDC, "Condoms for prevention of sexually transmitted diseases," *MMWR* 37, no. 9 (1988): 133–37.

19. J. S. Park, "The Effective Prevention of HIV by Female Condom (Femidon)" (International Conference on AIDS, August 7–12, 1994) (abstract PC0531), vol. 10 (2), 288.

20. M. A. Leeper, "Evaluation of the WPC-333 female condom barriers" (International Conference on AIDS, June 4–9, 1989) (abstract WDP 39), vol. 5, 749.

21. S. L. Coulter et al., "Low Particle Transmission across Polyurethane Condoms" (International Conference on AIDS, June 16–21, 1991) (abstract MC3022), vol. 7 (1), 303.

22. D. Hicks et al., "Inactivation of LAV/HTLV-III infected cultures of normal human lymphocytes by nonoxynol-9 in vitro," *Lancet* 2 (1985): 1422.

23. Winkelstein et al., "Sexual practices and risk," 321–25.

24. T. Quinn et al., "Human immunodeficiency virus infection among patients attending clinics for sexually transmitted diseases," *NEJM* 318, no. 4 (1988): 197–203; and W. Stamm et al., "The association between genital ulcer disease and acquisition of HIV infection in homosexual men," *JAMA* 260, no. 10 (September 9, 1988): 1429–33.

Chapter 4

1. D. Imagawa et al., "Human immunodeficiency virus type 1 infection in homosexual men who remain seronegative for prolonged periods," *NEJM* 320, no. 22 (June 1, 1989): 1458.

2. J. Groopman et al., "Lack of evidence of prolonged human immunodeficiency virus infection before antibody seroconversion," *Blood* 71 (1988): 1752–54.

3. J. Genesca et al., "What do Western blot indeterminate patterns for human immunodeficiency virus mean in EIA-negative blood donors?" *Lancet*, October 28, 1989.

4. CDC, "Interpretation and use of the Western blot assay for serodiagnosis of human immunodeficiency virus type 1 infections," *MMWR* 38:S-7 (July 28, 1989): 1–7.

5. CDC, "Update—Serologic testing for antibody to human immunodeficiency virus," *MMWR* 36 (1988): 833–40, 845.

6. K. Myer and S. Pauker, "Screening for HIV: can we afford the false-positive rate?" *NEJM* 317, no. 4 (July 23, 1987): 238–41.

7. N. Hessol et al., "Projections of the cumulative proportion of HIV-infected men who will develop AIDS [abstract]" (28th Interscience Conference on Antimicrobial Agents and Chemotherapy, Los Angeles, October 23–26, 1988), 170.

8. K-J. Lui et al., "A model-based estimate of the mean incubation period for AIDS in homosexual men," *Science* 240 (1988): 1333–35.

9. CDC, "Update—HIV-2 infection—United States," *MMWR* 38, no. 33 (August 25, 1989): 572–80.

10. N. Barry, "Screening for HIV infection: risks, benefits, and the burden of proof," *Law, Medicine, and Health Care* 14, no. 5–6 (December 1986): 259–67.

Chapter 5

1. P. D. Smith, moderator, "Gastrointestinal infections in AIDS," *AIM* 116 (1992): 63–77.

2. L. Young, "Treatable aspects of infection due to human immunodeficiency virus," *Lancet* 8574, no. 2 (December 1987): 1503–6.

3. R. Soave and W. Johnson, "*Cryptosporidium* and *Isospora belli* infections," *Journal of Infectious Diseases* 157, no. 2 (February 1988): 225–29.

4. L. Kaplan et al., "Treatment of patients with acquired immunodeficiency syndrome and association manifestations," *JAMA* 257, no. 10 (March 1987): 1367–74.

5. C. T. Leach et al., "A longitudinal study of cytomegalovirus infection in human immunodeficiency virus type-1 seropositive homosexual men: molecular epidemiology and association with disease progression," *Journal of Infectious Diseases* 170 (1994): 293–98.

6. J. Mulder et al., "Rapid and Simple PCR Assay for Quantitation of Human Immunodeficiency Virus Type 1 RNA Plasma: Application to Acute Retroviral Infection, *J. Clin. Microbiol.* 32, no. 2 (February 1994): 292–300.

7. D. Ho et al., "Rapid Turnover of Plasma Virions and CD4 Lymphocytes in HIV Infection," *Nature* 373 (January 1995): 123–26.

8. CDC, "Immunization of children infected with human immunodeficiency virus—supplementary ACIP statement," *MMWR* 37, no. 12 (April 1, 1988): 181–83.

9. CDC, "Hepatitis B vaccine: evidence confirming lack of AIDS transmission," *MMWR* 33 (1984): 685–87.

10. CDC, "Tuberculosis, final data—United States, 1986," *MMWR* 36, nos. 50, 51 (January 1, 1988): 817–20.

11. CDC, "Diagnosis and management of mycobacterial infection and disease in persons with human T-lymphotropic virus,

type III/lymphadenopathy-associated virus infection," *MMWR* 35 (1986): 448–52.

12. M. O'Sullivan, "Management of Women with AIDS" (AMFAR Conference, March 31–April 2, 1995).

13. M. Hoyt, "National Conference Examines HIV/AIDS in Women," *GMHC Treatment Issues* 9, no. 3 (March 1995): 1–3.

14. G. Gibbs et al. in H. Libman et al., *HIV Infection: A Clinical Manual* (Boston: Little, Brown, and Company, 1995), 394–422.

15. B. Spurrett et al., "Cervical dysplasia and HIV infection," *Lancet* 1:8579 (1988): 237–39.

16. A. Lifson et al., "The natural history of human immunodeficiency virus infection," *Journal of Infectious Diseases* 158, no. 6 (December 1988): 1364.

17. G. Friedland and R. Klein, "Transmission of the human immunodeficiency virus," *NEJM* 317, no. 18 (October 1987): 1125–35.

18. H. Minkoff, "Care of pregnant women infected with human immunodeficiency virus," *JAMA* 258, no. 19 (November 1987): 2714–17.

19. S. Katz et al., "Human immunodeficiency virus infection of newborns," *NEJM* 320, no. 25 (June 1989): 1687–89.

20. C. Walsh and S. Savona, "Hematologic findings in HIV infection," in G. Wormser et al., *AIDS—acquired immunodeficiency syndrome—and other manifestations of HIV infection* (Park Ridge, NJ: Noyes Publications, 1987), 783–95.

21. L. Mass, *Medical Answers About AIDS*, 3rd ed. (New York: Gay Men's Health Crisis, 1987).

22. W. F. Jekot and D. W. Purdy, "Treating HIV/AIDS patients with anabolic steroids: A retrospective study," *AIDS Patient Care* (April 1993): 68–74.

23. B. Gingell, "Nutrition and AIDS," *GMHC Treatment Issues* (Gay Men's Health Crisis Medical Information Department) 1, no. 1 (November 27, 1987): 4–7.

24. A. Beneson, ed., *Control of Communicable Diseases in Man* (Washington, D.C.: American Public Health Association, 1985), 392–94.

25. Kaplan et al., "Treatment of patients," 1367–74.

26. C. Metroka et al., "Successful chemoprophylaxis for *Pneumocystis carinii* pneumonia with dapsone in patients with

AIDS and ARC" (Third International Conference on AIDS, June 1–5, 1987, Washington, D.C.) (TH P 231), 202.

27. CDC, "Recommendations for prophylaxis against *Pneumocystis carinii* pneumonia for adults and adolescents infected with HIV," *MMWR* 41 (1992): 1–12.

28. M. J. Fisher et al., "Atovaquone as prophylaxis against *Pneumocystis carinii* pneumonia" (letter), *Journal of Infectious Diseases* 28 (1994): 103–4.

29. CDC, "Guidelines for prophylaxis against *Pneumocystis carinii* pneumonia for persons infected with human immunodeficiency virus," *MMWR* 38 (1989): S-5.

30. E. Camus et al., "Effect of corticosteroids on the incidence of adverse cutaneous reactions to trimethoprim-sulfamethazole during treatment of AIDS-associated *Pneumocystis carinii* pneumonia," *Clin. Infect. Dis.* 18 (1994): 319–23.

31. A. Carr et al., "Low-dose trimethoprim-sulfamethazole prophylaxis for toxoplasmic encephalitis," *AIM* 117 (1992): 106–11.

32. J. Gallant et al., "Prophylaxis for opportunistic infections in patients with HIV infection," *NEJM* 120, no. 11 (June 1994): 932–44.

33. D. Gilden, "Ganciclovir Approved to Prevent CMV," *GMHC Treatment Issues,* 9, no. 11 (Nov. 1995): 3.

34. F. Gordin and H. Masur, "Prophylaxis of *Mycobacterium avium* complex bacteremia in patients with AIDS," *Clin. Infect. Dis.* 18 (1994): 5223–26.

35. M. Hirsch, "Azidothymidine," *Journal of Infectious Diseases* 157, no. 3 (March 1988): 427–31.

36. M. Fischl et al., "Efficacy of azidothymidine (AZT) in the treatment of patients with AIDS and AIDS-related complex," *NEJM* 317, no. 4 (July 23, 1987): 185–91.

37. M. Fischl et al., "Prolonged zidovudine therapy in patients with AIDS and advanced AIDS-related complex," *JAMA* 262, no. 17 (November 3, 1989): 2405–10.

38. T. Creagh-Kirk et al., "Survival experience among patients with AIDS receiving zidovudine," *JAMA* 260, no. 20 (1988): 3009.

39. E. Dournon et al., "Effects of zidovudine in 365 consecutive patients with AIDS or AIDS-related complex," *Lancet* (December 3, 1988): 1297.

40. P. Volberding, "Initiation of Antiretroviral Therapy in HIV Infection: A Review of Interstudy Consistencies," *Journal of the Acquired Immune Deficiency Syndrome* 7, no. 2 (1994): S12–S23.

41. P. Volberding et al., "Safety and efficacy of zidovudine in asymptomatic HIV-infected individuals with less than 500 CD4 + cells/mm³," *NEJM* 322 (1990): 941–49.

42. M. Fischl et al., "The safety and efficacy of zidovudine (AZT) in the treatment of patients with mildly symptomatic HIV infection—a double-blind, placebo-controlled trial," *AIM* 112 (1990): 727–37.

43. D. Richman et al., "The toxicity of azidothymidine (AZT) in the treatment of patients with AIDS and AIDS-related complex," *NEJM* 317, no. 4 (July 23, 1987), 192–97.

44. C. Debouck, "The HIV-1 protease as a therapeutic target for AIDS," *AIDS Research & Human Retroviruses* 8, no. 2 (February 1992): 153–64.

45. H. Moh et al., "The Patterns of Specific Mutations in HIV 1 Protease That Confer Resistance to a Panel of Protease Inhibitors" (Second National Conference on Human Retroviruses and Related Infections, 1995) (abstract 188), 89.

46. R. Loftus et al., "Protease Inhibitors: Where are they NOW," *GMHC Treatment Issues* 9, no. 1 (January 1995) 1–7.

47. J. A. Kovacs et al., "Immunologic enhancement in HIV-infected patients with intermittent interleukin-2 therapy" (33rd ICAAC, 1993) (abstract 1141).

48. Kaplan et al., "Treatment of patients," 1367–74.

Chapter 7

1. "Anti-gay violence, victimization and defamation in 1988," National Gay and Lesbian Task Force, Washington, D.C., 1988.

2. "Education and foster care of children infected with human T-lymphotropic virus, type III/lymphadenopathy-associated virus," *MMWR* 34 (August 30, 1985): 517–21.

3. K. Fraser, "Someone at school has AIDS—a guide to developing policies for students and school staff members who are infected with HIV," National Association of State Boards of Education, 1012 Cameron St., Alexandria, VA 22314, 1989.

4. M. Barnes, D. Greenberg, and L. Pinsky, "Providing high-quality, low-cost legal services to people with AIDS—an antidiscrimination law project," *AIDS Care* 1, no. 3 (1989): 297–306.

5. *Estelle v Gamble,* 429 US 97 (1976).

6. N. Gilmore et al., "International travel and AIDS," *AIDS* 3, suppl. 1 (1989): S2229.

ABOUT THE AUTHORS

LAURA PINSKY is the director of the Columbia Gay Health Advocacy Project. Ms. Pinsky is also a psychotherapist at the Columbia University Health Service Counseling and Psychology Service and in private practice in New York City. PAUL HARDING DOUGLAS was the former co-director of the Columbia Gay Health Advocacy Project. He was a faculty member of the Cornell University Medical College and a senior research associate at the Cornell AIDS Clinical Trial Unit. They have based this book on ten years' work counseling and lecturing about AIDS at Columbia and consulting for the Gay Men's Health Crisis and other organizations. They are also the authors of a book on treatments and early intervention for AIDS and HIV disease entitled *The Essential HIV Treatment Fact Book*.

Paul Douglas died of AIDS in July 1995.